Timber's Story

Living with a Spooky Lady from her Guide Dogs point of view

To Alan
with love
Angela Brigenshaw
April 2018.

By

Angela Brigenshaw

Timber's Story

First paperback edition printed 2017 in the United Kingdom

ISBN 978-1-910815-02-1

A catalogue record for this book is available from the British Library.

Published by Herkimer Publishing
www.herkimerpublishing.com

Design by Mystic Mouse Design

Dedication

For Timber, in memory for all the help he gave me and wonderful days we spent together.

For my husband David, without his help and support this book would not have been written.

For the work done by British Wireless for the Blind Fund in helping to provide visually impaired people with the companionship of radio. For further details please see:

http://www.blind.org.uk/

About the Author

Angela was diagnosed with Retinitis Pigmentosa, a degenerative condition resulting in progressively worsening tunnel vision, in 1977. This condition can in certain circumstances result in total blindness but Angela has been lucky in that she still has some sight. It wasn't until 1994 that Angela received her first guide dog, Owen. In 2007 Angela met her second guide dog Timber.

Angela's life has taken her in many directions including Spiritualism. Angela travels around the South East of England demonstrating her mediumship. She is happily married to her husband David, who is also a working medium. The couple live in Kent.

Foreword and Acknowledgements.

Firstly, I would like to say 'Thank You' for purchasing this book.

I hit upon the idea of writing Timber's Story when he passed away in December 2015. After I'd put a status on Facebook about Timber's passing, I was amazed at the number of people who told me how much they loved Timber and made comments about his character and what he used to get up to. This is what gave me the idea of writing a book about my life with Timber as seen through his eyes.

One of my aims in writing this book is that I would like to make a donation to Guide Dogs (Charity number 209617) by way of saying Thank You to them for the valuable work that they do and for bringing Timber into my life.

While you are reading Timber's Story, you may think that he was always mischievous and naughty. He certainly had his moments but he was also a good, loyal working guide dog. I wouldn't want to put off anybody who is thinking of applying for a guide dog. I would say go for it, even if you have never thought about doing so. The rewards will outweigh any 'teething problems' you may encounter. Don't forget that every single dog acts, behaves, and has emotions and feelings just like you and me.

That's what makes them all so unique and Timber taught me this very valuable lesson.

You can follow Timber's Story on:-

Facebook – Timber's Story, Living with a Spooky Lady from her Guide Dogs Point of view.

Web page – **www.timbersstory.com**

E-mail – **timbersstory@zoho.com**

I would also like to thank:

Wigmore Veterinary Surgery, 392 Maidstone Road, Rainham, Kent ME8 0JA, telephone 01634 388045, for looking after Timber and ministering to him at the end;

Jonathan Cooke for his kind permission to use some of the photographs reproduced in this book. You can contact him on www.jccreate.com or by E-mail at jcphotocooke@gmail.com;

Guide Dogs for the Blind for permission to reproduce pictures from Timber's Pupdate bulletin;

Becky Smith, a great friend of Timber and me. Please contact her on www.pegasoanimalhealing.co.uk to learn more about animal healing.

Timber's Story

Living with a Spooky Lady from her Guide Dogs point of view

Contents

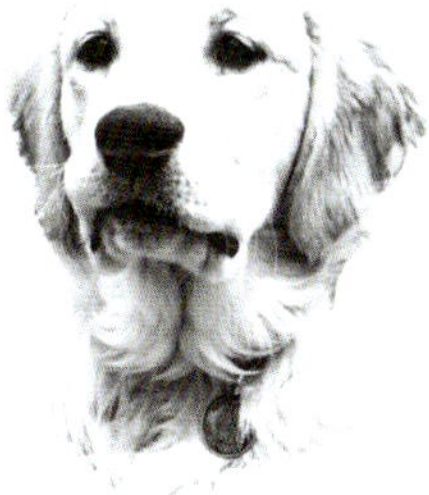

Chapter One

My Early Years

It has gone quiet. My mistress has gone off to bed so I'm thinking to myself 'it's now or never'. I've been watching her every move as she works away at her computer day after day and it doesn't look too difficult to get up on the chair and do the same.

Right, here goes. I jump up onto the chair and it starts to move all over the place; help! I manage to stop it swivelling around, phew! Now, looking at the screen and this thing she calls a keyboard, I have to try and remember how to turn it on. I don't have delicate paws you see, so I gingerly reach out and press this button to turn the screen on. Oops, careful I don't push it too hard as the screen starts to move back. The screen comes to life and then I start to look around it to see how I can start typing a document. Ahh there it is, so I press it and up comes a blank document to enable me to write. Here goes.

First, I'm going to introduce myself. My name is Timber and I'm a very handsome Golden Retriever, even if I say so myself. I was born on the seventh of June, 2005. I was chosen to do a special job, helping people who cannot see very well or who are completely blind.

My father's name was Windsor and he was a stud for Guide Dogs. I don't know my mother's name, she was just mum to me. I was one of a litter and stayed with my brothers and sisters until I was eight weeks old. This was when I was placed with a couple called Sid and Trish who were known as Puppy Raisers.

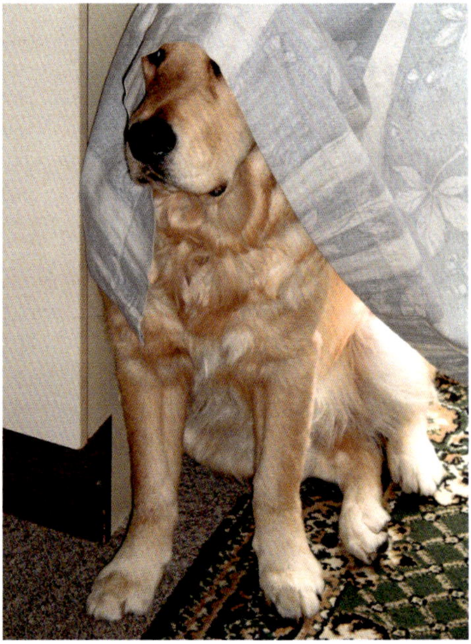

Unsuccessfully trying to hide!

I was very frightened at first when I was taken away from my mother and siblings. I wanted to be with them; not with these strangers. Sid and Trish made such a fuss of me by giving me lots of cuddles to make me feel at home and there were other dogs around. Brooke, who was another trainee guide dog, and Jazz the German Shepherd. Jazz was Sid and Trish's own pet dog.

Sid and Trish had looked after many other guide dog puppies before me and they had a lot of experience in taking take care of us. They were expecting another puppy who was younger than me; his name was Arnie. I heard them say that I was the youngest puppy they'd had up to that time and when Arnie came along I would help him and show him who was boss. I really loved playing with the other dogs, especially at tug of war!

I was taken everywhere Sid and Trish went. They took me on buses, in cars, on trains, to parties, everywhere so that I would get used to sights, sounds and smells. They also told me off if I did something naughty, that happened often as I used to get into scrapes. I was very mischievous but I was also loving toward others. I didn't show some of the Retriever's traits of wilfulness then; that came later.

I didn't like anyone playing with my toys. Not only did I have my own, I used to pinch the other dogs' toys too and wouldn't let them have them back. There were times when you would see me walking around with a toy or ball in my mouth, doing absolutely nothing with it. I didn't chew it, I just carried it to stop the other dogs from getting hold of it!

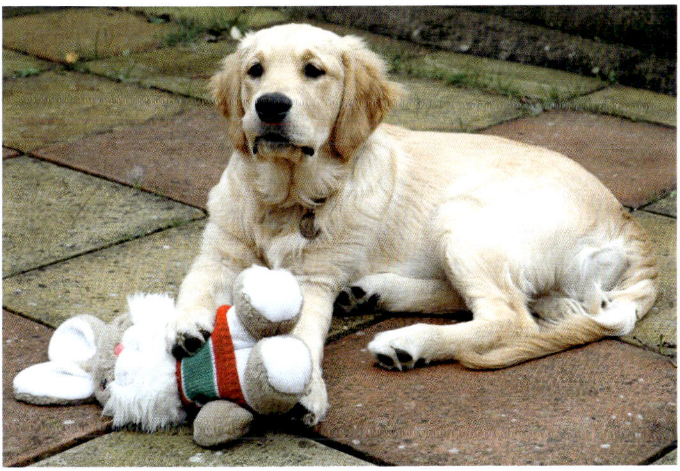

Guarding mine and the other's toys!

When I used to go out for walks, I would go with either Sid who walked faster or with Trish who walked more slowly. This showed me that not everybody walks at the same speed and that I had to get used to different peoples' walking speeds. They took me to places with lifts and some of these had glass all round and I could look at what was going on down below me. Even the stairs with gaps didn't faze me.

There was one place they took me to, that was the vet's. I wasn't too sure of the Vet and his staff at first. I didn't like it when I felt a sharp prick go into my skin. I would get weighed, then I got pulled, prodded, had my mouth opened to check my teeth and gums. But eventually I got used to it and didn't mind going there as I knew what to expect. There was the added bonus of getting a treat before leaving the surgery. That made it all worthwhile.

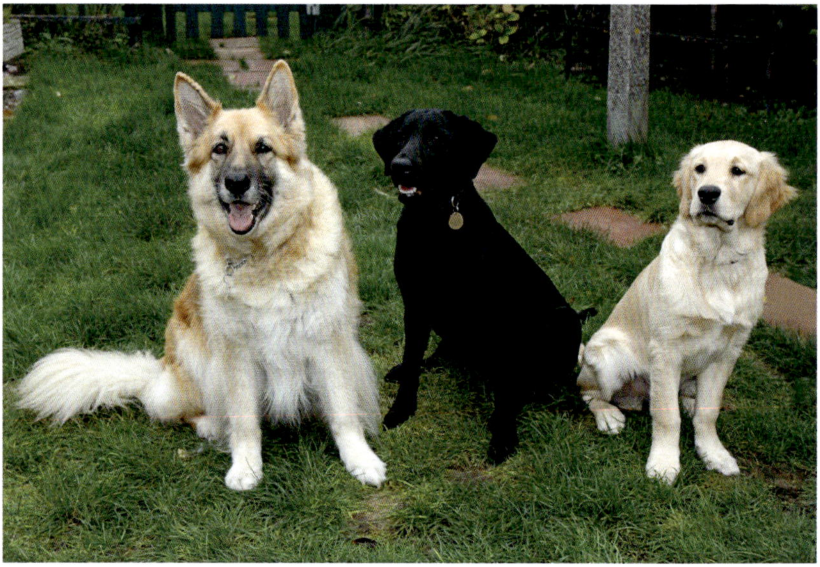

Jazz, Brooke and Me.

I eventually settled into a lovely routine going out for walks and playing with the other dogs, especially with Jazz with whom I built a close friendship. I often used to go to her for a cuddle or just to let her know that I was around when the others were making her life a misery, especially Arnie. He used to tease her rotten.

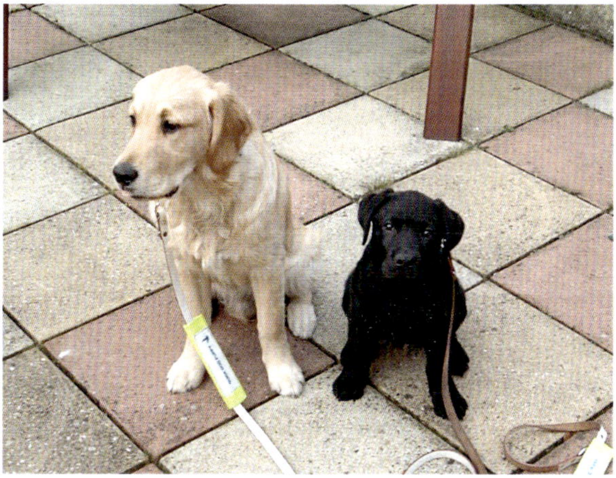

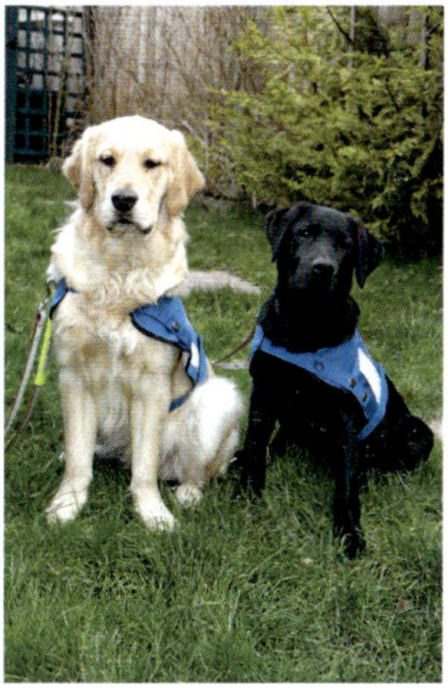

Arnie and me (left). Arnie and I wearing our Blue Coats (right)

I was about a year old and was well behaved. Sid and Trish took Arnie and me with them to rattle their collecting tins in the High Street or somewhere. Sid and Trish were very keen fundraisers for Guide Dogs and raised a lot of money for them. I really loved all the attention that I got, especially when Arnie and I were chosen to receive a cheque from Andrex. We even got our picture into the local newspapers; fame! Sid and Trish were asked to visit the local school where the children had been fundraising for Guide Dogs and they too presented us with a cheque. After the pictures had been taken, we went round to the different classrooms to meet all the children to say thank you; they made a lot of fuss of us and gave us lots of cuddles. I do like my cuddles!

Then one day someone came to talk to Sid and Trish about me. This person was saying that as I was coming up to fourteen months old; it was time for me to leave and go somewhere else. 'What! Leave? I can't leave, I like it here'. It was about a week later when a lady came and collected me with all of my belongings and put me into the back of her van. I was frightened again as I didn't know what was happening. I just wanted to be back with my friends.

We arrived at a strange place and I was put into a kennel. I'd never been in a kennel before, and it was a strange experience for me. I could see the other dogs but I couldn't get to them. I felt so alone. A lady kept coming up to me and talking to me all the time. I eventually found out that her name was Katrina and that she was a guide dog trainer who would develop my skills still further.

I was taken out of my kennel so that I could go outside to do my 'spending', that's spending a penny to you humans! I had to keep walking up and down until I had 'spent'. This could be frustrating for me as I might not want to go at any particular moment! Mind you, life wasn't that bad in the kennels. I did have a lot of playmates to keep me company and yes, I was still carrying a ball in my mouth.

What my training involved was learning to walk in a straight line, to 'come over' and 'in' to avoid obstacles which I practiced on the obstacle course at the training centre. Some of you may be wondering whether I can see the different colours of traffic lights. The answer is 'no.' I was told what to do about this when receiving more training later on. I had to learn my left from my right, and that can be a bit confusing at times I can tell you! Then one day, I felt a change happening to me. I was used to wearing a blue coat that said I was a puppy guide dog. Now I began to wear something much heavier with a handle, and Katrina started to train me differently with this thing called a harness. It was made of brown leather with a reflective yellow panel on the front and had a funny shaped metal handle with a leather grip. I got to learn that as soon as the harness was placed over my head I had to work and that my play time was over. It got to the stage where I was so used to wearing it that I raised my head up to make it easier for the harness to go over my head.

I loved going out working but there were times when I said 'enough is enough' and just plonked myself down, especially if we were anywhere near a café. Then down I went to have a snooze!

After a while, I was being moved again! This time I was going into my final stage of training. I was introduced to a new lady called Sam, who was known as a Mobility Instructor. I didn't like this bit and I played up; I just couldn't get settled into the new routine, which seemed too much like hard work. Not only was I with another new lady, I was staying in a house with a boarder family. I was lucky though as they had a pet dog. I was even luckier that he had so many toys. I wasn't going to let him play with them. To make sure, I stood guard over the toy box.

I loved it when I got a lot of praise. On hearing this I used to puff out my chest and I found my tail used to go up and wag like mad. I felt so proud.

The next part of training involved travelling on the underground in London. When we got to the London station, I saw a great many birds. They were called pigeons, and they were everywhere! Another thing that sticks in my mind about London is that it's noisy!!

I really didn't like heavy traffic and I felt so scared of the big vehicles. They were noisy and I could smell all the fumes; Yuk. That was when I showed my stubborn side. I was not going to do what I was told, no way. The trouble was, the more stubborn I became the more they made me do what I didn't want to so I thought I might just as well get used to it and do as I was told.

I didn't realise at the time that I had such an important job to do. How could I? I was a puppy.

Oops, better stop now, I can hear my mistress moving around, so I'd better get things closed down and vacate this chair quick! Phew, just managed it. I'm back into my bed quick and straight to sleep. The next thing I'm being woken to be let out to spend. No, I'm tired, I want to stay here. But out I go, all the same!

Later in the day I overhear my mistress say that she will have to change the computer chair. Somehow there are hairs all over it and it doesn't seem safe. She soon changed it for a more solid chair that didn't move about so much. I liked that idea.

I'd sleep all day if it wasn't for my mistress wanting to go out. So, up I get and I do what I have to do.

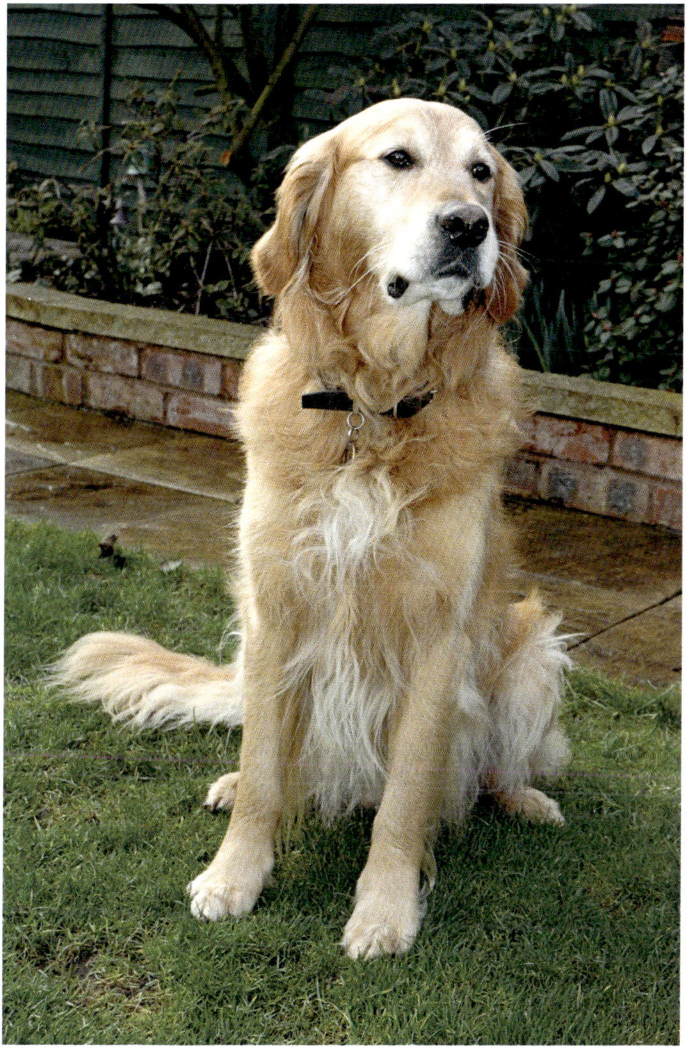

Looking so handsome!

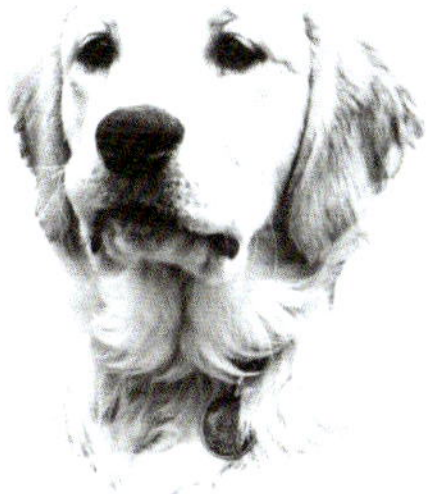

Chapter 2

Meeting Angela and our training together

Right, I feel a lot better now and this chair feels a lot safer. At least I'm not swivelling around on it. Now where were we? Ahh yes, training with Sam.

The day came when Sam turned to me and said 'right Timber, you're ready to leave us'. Leave us, I thought, why, where am I going now?

By this time another lady had come into my life. Her name was Lesley. It was in December 2006 when she put me into the back of her van and I was taken to another house. She pulled up onto the drive and then let me out of the back. Lesley said 'Right Timber, I want you to be a good boy and be on your best behaviour'. We walked up to the front door and she rang the bell. After a short while another lady opened the door and greeted Lesley. She then opened the door wide so that we could go into the house. I did notice that she had tears in her eyes and I thought 'hey up, what's going on?' Did she know something I didn't? Anyway, we entered the house and went into the living room. There was a lot of talking going on and I wasn't really taking much notice. I wanted to wander off and explore but Lesley wouldn't let me. I was looking around the room, it looked nice. As I couldn't wander off, I started to look at this lady, I thought 'she doesn't look bad, she seems nice'. I then discovered her name was Angela. She began to stroke my head. I liked that, but I was still curious as to why I was there.

After talking for a while, Lesley told Angela to take me out into the garden to 'spend'. This was so that I didn't stop to relieve myself whilst we were out, which might cause Angela to wonder what was going on with me. After that, Lesley showed Angela how to put the harness, which had now been changed from brown to white, on me and clip it underneath my tummy. Then Angela held the handle and walked me out of the door with Lesley following. I could sense straight away from the way she was holding the handle that she was very nervous. My nose was on overdrive because of all the different smells that were around me. Lesley told Angela to take me to the edge of the kerb and make me sit to wait for the next command. Lesley told Angela to find left and we continued like this walking along four different roads until we arrived back at Angela's house.

When we got back indoors my harness was taken off, Lesley told Angela to give me a lot of praise and to take me back outside to 'spend' again. The reason for this is that the motion of walking can cause my bowels to start moving so I need an opportunity to relieve myself. I still had my lead on, so Lesley unclipped it and said 'there you go boy, welcome to your new home'. I immediately went on a tour of the rooms to investigate my new house. There were only two rooms downstairs, the living room and kitchen/diner. When I came back, Angela called me over and I sat beside her. She then got down onto the floor to my level and we just looked into each other's eyes. I placed my paw onto her arm and then gave her a lick on her face and said 'you'll do'. I felt it was a special moment between the two of us. After a short while Lesley and I left and I didn't see Angela again until twelfth January 2007.

It was a Friday. Lesley put my bowls, grooming kit, bed and my feed into the back of her car and then I jumped into the boot where there was a grille to stop me climbing into the back seats. As we were driving along, I began to recognise where I was going, especially when we pulled up outside Angela's house, my new home. Angela was very happy to see me and I her. Lesley sat down and filled out the necessary paperwork. She explained to Angela about my feeding, and the spending routines. She told her that a taxi would be picking her up with me on the following Monday to begin our training in Maidstone, the county town of Kent. When Lesley left us alone, I kept wondering where she had gone and kept looking out of the window and wondering when she was going to pick me up to take me home. I didn't fully realise that this new house was going to be my home now and that Angela and I were going to have a special bond together.

I think it's time I told you a little bit about Angela.

Angela was born in July 1956 to a single mother. Her Father didn't want to know anything about her or have any involvement with her during her formative years. Angela's Mother eventually married when she was still a baby. Her new husband said he would accept Angela as one of his own, but this turned out to be the worst thing that could have happened to her. Her step-father was a very abusive man who was very free with his hands. When Angela was three years old, he beat her so badly that she became deaf. She grew up moving from place to place; never settling down anywhere. After so much violence from her husband, her Mother decided to leave him and ended up in a hostel for homeless mums and their children in West Malling, Kent. Angela grew up making the best of her situation and eventually met and married her first husband. They had 3 children together. After 20 years, their marriage unfortunately broke down.

Angela left her first husband and met and married her second, which proved to be a great mistake. She left him after seven years of marriage and moved to where she was living now. She had been living alone for 3 years until I came on the scene.

I did find out that Angela had already had a previous guide dog named Owen, who was a Yellow Labrador. He was five when she had him but Angela had to give him up due to the behaviour of her second husband and her terrible living conditions. She felt it wasn't fair to put Owen through these troubles. She was heartbroken when she gave him to a friend of hers but knew it was for the best.

Angela made a great fuss of me on our first day together to help me settle in. She talked to me for a while and then I settled down for a kip, it had been a busy day. It was just before Angela wanted to go to bed that she took me outside to have my spend. It was dark and I'd decided that I was not having any of that I can tell you! I could tell she was feeling rather tense and all I kept getting in my ear walking up and down was 'busy, busy', with her holding the torch, flashing about me and I'd already decided that I wasn't going to go. I can't imagine what the neighbours must have thought about hearing a voice saying 'busy, busy' and seeing this torch waving all over the place, hee, hee! After a good while of nothing happening, we went back indoors. She got me settled into my bed and went up to bed herself, leaving the door open. What I had not realised was that Angela was deaf and in both ears too thanks to her step-father.

When morning came, I was lying out on the hall landing and I didn't go to Angela. She got up and went into the bathroom, then walked into the back bedroom. Then I heard 'Oh no Timber, what the hell have you done', as she was scraping my deposit from the bottom of her foot. I just went and disappeared; too right!

After her shower, we went downstairs and she took me out to relieve myself properly, then we got ready to go out on our first day of training together. It was whilst Angela was opening the curtain across the front door that she stood on another 'package' I'd left for her. That got her even more mad. I thought I had better disappear until she calmed down.

The taxi arrived to collect us, Angela got in and beckoned me to sit between her legs which I did. I always made sure that my tail was safely tucked in, as I didn't want it to be caught in the door. That makes me wince just thinking of it.

We were taken to The Hilton Hotel in Maidstone. I met another playmate there called Wispa with her mistress Anne who was totally blind. The worst thing about it was that I wasn't allowed to go running around the room to have a play; it wasn't fair. I got bored with just lying there, waiting for something to happen. In the afternoon we did do things when we went out. Angela was being given different instructions on how to make certain signals and give different commands to me when stopping at kerbs or crossing roads. Everything was done in straight lines, giving me commands with 'back' whilst slapping her thigh, that meant turning round and going back the way we had come. When we came up to a set of traffic lights or a pedestrian crossing, I would have to wait for Angela to give me the command to cross the road when the lights changed as I can't see colours in the range from green to red. Angela therefore had to rely on her hearing to know when the pedestrian light had changed or the traffic had stopped. If Angela needed to cross a very busy road, she would drop my harness down on my back and get out a card that read something like 'Can you please help'. This then enables anyone to help her across the road with no danger to herself.

We were working really well together. It was on the second week that I really chanced my paw. I'd had enough of all this working and being told what to do so I decided to play up. We were walking through Maidstone High Street and Angela was giving me commands to find and take her to a particular store. I thought ‘nope, I’m not going’ and proceeded to ignore her. She gave me other commands and I still ignored her. Angela was told to stop and to give the command of ‘sit’ to me. I duly sat, all innocent like. Lesley told me off! Angela was in a state, she became tearful and told Lesley she didn’t want to have me or any other guide dog, full stop.

Lesley suggested that we finish for the day and took us home. She talked to Angela saying that there would be days like this and that she would have to show me who was boss. After Lesley had gone, Angela picked up the phone to talk to her daughter Clair and told her about what a horrible day it had been and what she was thinking of doing. Clair must have told her not to give in, just keep going. After a good night’s sleep she was a different person the next morning. A new determination had set in and boy didn’t I know it!

I was still having trouble settling in, I still made a mess on the floor but eventually it did get sorted and I didn’t do it inside the house anymore, much to Angela’s relief!

The best thing that I really enjoyed was when we went to Mote Park in Maidstone for the free run. I was pulling and pulling desperately to get off the lead and run, to be free! There were so many other dogs out there. Before Angela could let me go, she had to make me lie down and do this obedience thing. I had to lie down, sit and stay. When Angela walked away I still had to sit there and not move. I tolerated it as I just wanted to get going, then she said the magic words, one, two, three GO!

Whoopee, I was free, running like anything with Wispa, jumping, rolling over the grass and finding other dogs to play with. I was just getting going when I heard this whistle and a call from Angela to come back. I went running back and she gave me some lovely treats for being a good boy. She told me to sit again and then gave the command 'go on boy'. I got into a right clan of dogs, there must have been about 12 of us all sniffing each other's bottoms and one even tried to 'hump' me, I was just standing there and thinking this was such fun.

After some time running around the park getting absolutely filthy and feeling ecstatic, I was called back again and my leash was clipped on. We were then taken back to the hotel, exhausted.

Angela and I soon got settled into a routine, me deciding when I was going to 'spend', and Angela getting frustrated with me; we did work together well, I let her think it anyway.

After about three weeks, there seemed to be some excitement in the air. The taxi didn't come and pick us up as usual but someone else came with Lesley who looked important. It turned out that he was the Manager of Maidstone Guide Dogs who had come to assess us to see if we qualified to work together permanently. There was also another man there with a camera taking pictures of us. The time came for us to go and do the final walk around to see if I was doing my job properly and to see if Angela was coping with having me on the harness.

I could tell that Angela was relieved when she heard that we had made it. Angela was told that the pictures that were being taken were to be put into a leaflet from which I found out that I was a sponsored dog. This meant that the public had sponsored me and followed my journey from a puppy till I was paired with a person with a sight problem. It's a fantastic way for Guide Dogs to raise money to enable more dogs to be trained like me.

Mind you, I did hear Angela being told that she had to continue to be a lot firmer with me. She was told not to allow me to stop and have a sniff at the wall or lamp post, especially when there were other dogs around. I tended to do a little double shuffle as if to say, 'hello, can I sniff you?' The answer to that from Angela was a definite NO!

It was from the day we qualified that we were completely on our own. We were left to do what we wanted and go where we wanted. Angela decided that she would go and visit her daughter Clair, who lived about 2 miles away. She placed the harness over my head and clipped on my lead. I suppose you are wondering why the lead as well? This is to enable Angela to have control when I play up, or there may be times when she has to let the harness down, for example if she is talking to someone, which then enables me to lay down on the ground. When we arrived at Clair's house, Angela knocked on the door and Clair answered but she looked a bit funny. She had this bump in front of her. I soon found out what this was all about. It was in February 2007 when Angela's mobile began to ring. She answered it in the dining room whilst looking out of the window. She started to cry when she finished talking to Clair and I came up and stood very close to her to give Angela a cuddle as if to say 'I'm here, what's up?'. Angela put her hand on top of my head and stroked it saying that we had a new addition to the family. Clair had just given birth to a baby girl whom they named Amelia.

It was later that week that Angela said we were going out to Maidstone which meant we had to go by bus. Angela was going to the KAB (Kent Association for the Blind) for computer lessons to hone her IT skills. The KAB do wonderful work for the blind and partially sighted people, far more than you could imagine.

I'd decided that I was going to show Angela who was boss again now that Lesley had left us. I had my chance that Wednesday, during the visit to the Maidstone KAB. Before leaving the house Angela took me outside to do my 'spend'. I made a feeble attempt at going and after a while Angela decided that I didn't want to go. We left the house and she told me to 'find the kerb' then told me to turn left to walk to another kerb at which she told me to sit. I got the command to cross the road and I knew we always went right so I proceeded to take her that way. She made me stop and sit and then gave the command to do it properly, so back we went. 'Oh well', I thought, 'I will get her on the next one'. On we went so I thought, right, I'm going to go up this street instead of going to the kerb. I knew where I wanted to go but she stopped me, told me off and we had to go back to the kerb again. I just kept her going like this all the time and then, when we got to where we needed to be to catch the bus, I just took her into the bushes. I'd had enough of her telling me off, and I wanted to get my own back!

I made several attempts to take her in a different way to the way she wanted to go, then 'oh dear', I wanted to do my spending. That was it, I was going and I didn't care what she thought. This got her into a flap; yes it was working, I was the boss.

We had no sooner arrived at the KAB centre when another dog came into the room. I wasn't going to listen to Angela when she said 'sit'. I wanted to play with my new friend. However, Angela had the upper hand and I had to do as I was told although not for long or so I thought.

After Angela had finished her computer lessons, we got ready to return home. What I didn't know was that Lesley was waiting in the reception area for her. They greeted each other and stood talking for a while. I hadn't realised that Angela had phoned Lesley explaining what I had been up to and she had come to collect us and take us into Maidstone town. We started working together and then Lesley told Angela to take me into the High Street. Again I decided I wasn't going to listen and went to take her another way and not only that, cross the road without stopping at the kerb. Lesley made Angela stop and tell me off. We went back the way we had come along the High Street then stopped and started again. I was getting everything wrong. I was picking up on Angela's anxieties through the harness. Then it all became too much for Angela as she became upset and flustered and began to cry. Lesley stopped the lesson and we went home. I could hear Lesley telling Angela that things like this were bound to happen at first. I was testing her to see how far I could go. It really was a battle of wills and she had to show me who the leader of the pack was.

We got home and Angela totally ignored me for the rest of the day apart from taking me out to spend and feeding me. It was early evening when I heard her talking to one of her friends saying that she was going to give me up as she couldn't cope with having me around and behaving the way I was. That really got me thinking about the way I was behaving. It was about time I started to behave myself. Although I was still only a puppy, I was 18 months old and qualified 6 months earlier than normal as I was very good during my training. It was me being so wilful thinking I knew best that got me into trouble. Angela couldn't relax with me for a while as she kept wondering what I was going to do next.

I loved it at night times when Angela went up to bed. Before we went upstairs, Angela would take me outside and I would relieve myself. Before she got into bed, she would make a huge fuss of me then I'd be happy to settle down till the morning.

One night, at about two in the morning, I was woken up by something entering the bedroom where we were. I went to Angela and tried rousing her as I was unsure of what it was I was seeing, but all I got from her was a mumbled 'Timber, go back to bed'. I later found out from listening to one of her friends who visited us a couple of days later that Angela was a special lady. I will try and explain this about her. Angela is able to communicate with the Spirit world as a Medium. Spirits come to her and I know this as I've seen them! Oh trust me to pick a strange one for my mistress, but I wouldn't change her for the world, she is so loving to me and I feel we have a strong connection.

Now to make it even more interesting. Angela started to take me to Church – boring. On our first trip together to a Church where Angela was going to demonstrate her mediumship, she sat me down beside her whilst she sat down in front of an audience. After a while I decided to go to sleep. All of a sudden I heard a lot of laughter at which I shot my head up wondering what was going on and what all the fuss was about. Apparently, Angela was giving someone a message and just at the critical moment, I started growling in my sleep and everyone thought it was a Spirit growling. I was so glad to be the centre of attention!

There were times when Angela was feeling very lonely during our early days together. She'd tell me how she was feeling and that she had nobody to talk to. It was while she was talking to me that I got up from the floor where I was lying and put my front two paw's on the settee and then placed one on her shoulder and gave her a cuddle. This really cheered her up and made her laugh.

We still had some teething problems but gradually Angela began to relax with me and we began to work better together. There were still some issues with regards to my messing on the floor. Angela solved that problem by not allowing me to come upstairs anymore. I missed going upstairs and waking her up at six every morning. I used to go to her room and put my head on the bed and thump it up and down, enough for her to know that it was me!

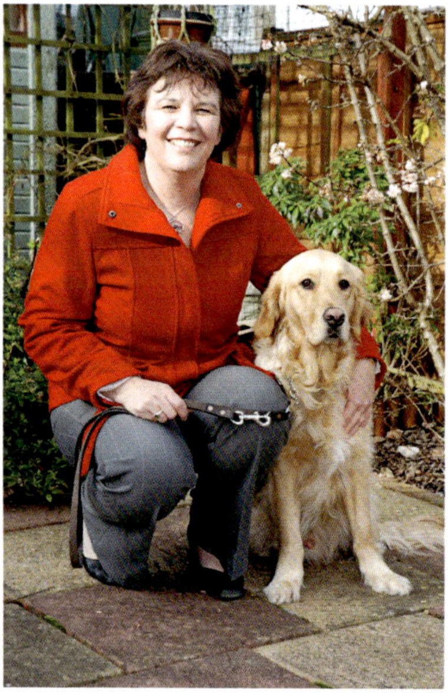

Angela and I on our qualifying day

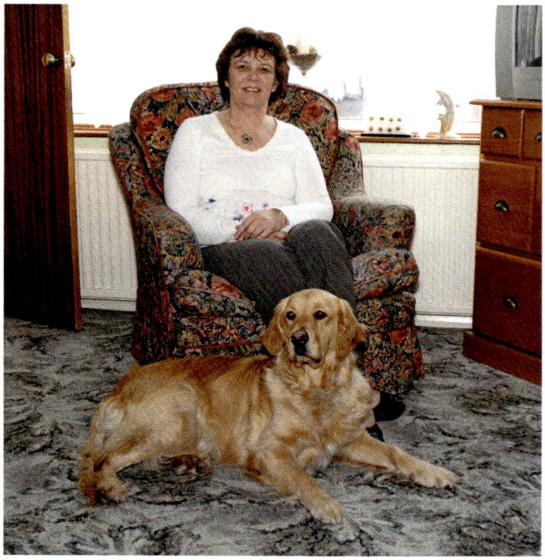

Family picture

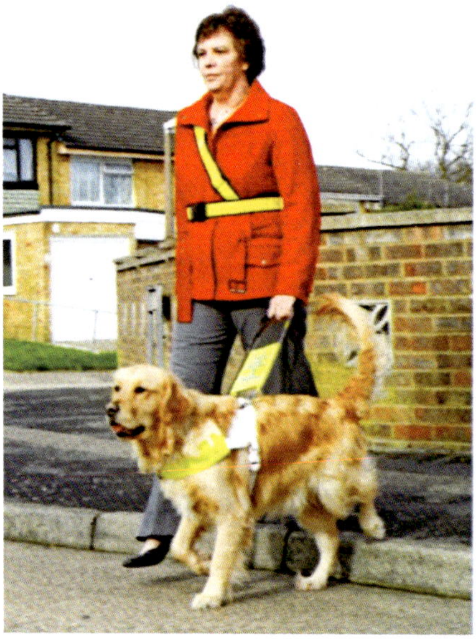

Angela and Me doing our qualifying walk

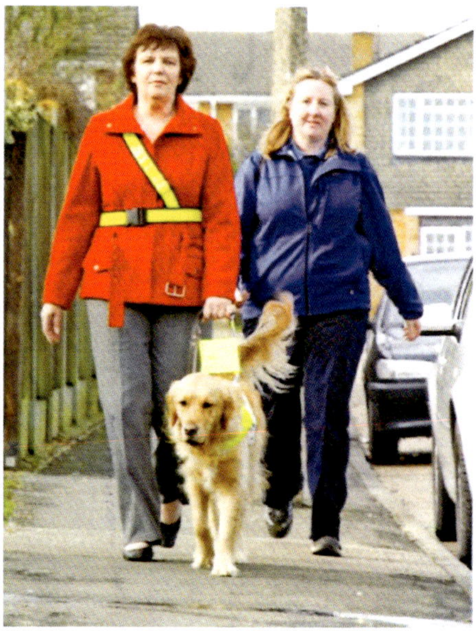

Our Trainer, Lesley walking behind us

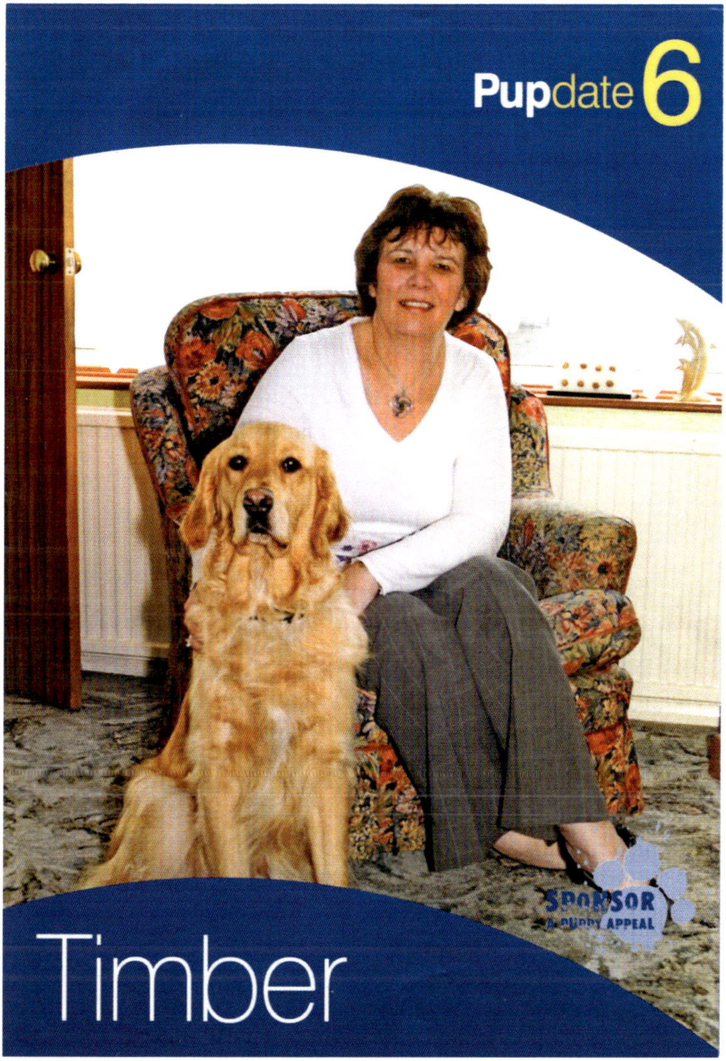

This is a copy of Pupdate for all those who sponsor a Guide Dog; giving information of the guide dogs progress and eventual pairing with a visually impaired client.

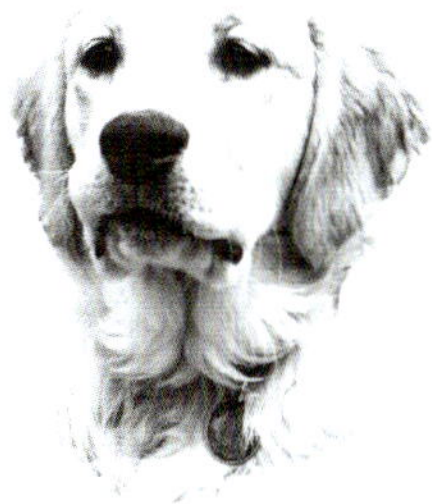

Chapter 3

Settling In

After a period of getting myself sorted, being told off about messing on the floor in the house and Angela phoning Lesley at Guide Dogs for help and guidance, I started to get the hang of things. I was staying. I also knew who was in charge – Angela. She was the leader of the pack.

I did wonder why I was paired up with Angela as she didn't look blind. She could still see me when I was being naughty and I got the answer one day when one of her friend's visited her.

Her friend Michelle came round for a coffee and a chat. I was always keen to go to the door to see who was there and if they would make a fuss of me, but Angela told me to 'stay' in my bed, so down I went, sulking.

When Michelle asked Angela why she had a guide dog; this is what she said:

I was nearly 21 when I decided that it was time I learned to drive. I was coming up for my driving test when the instructor asked me to read the number plate on the car in front. I struggled with it and missed some letters so the instructor advised me to go and have an eye test as I might need glasses

I went to the opticians and had the eye test. When he had finished examining my eyes, he turned to me and said there was something about my eyes he didn't like the look of. He said he was going to refer me to Moorfields Eye Hospital in London.

Mum and I went to Moorfields in September 1977. We were called into the consulting room and there were all these people standing there. We were introduced to them; they were students and doctors training under Professor Jay who was an eminent Eye Surgeon.

I was sent to different departments to undergo tests and I had a dye injected into my arm so that they could take pictures of the back of my eyes. After quite a few hours I was sent back upstairs to see the Professor for my results. This was the day that was to change my life forever.

When I was called in, the Professor explained to me what was going on with my eyes. He gave my condition a name, it was Retinitis Pigmentosa; RP for short. It was his next words that shook me to the core. 'I'm afraid that it's not good news, you are going blind. You could lose your sight sometime in the next 25 years or you could go blind overnight. What you have is tunnel vision. This condition is rare and is hereditary; which means you can pass it onto your children. I'd advise you to think seriously about whether you should start a family.

As you can imagine I was in shock and wondering how was I going to tell my husband and family. More importantly, what were we going to do about having children? We did go ahead with the family; I'm happy to say that none of the children have the condition.

I have Timber to help me around obstacles that are out of my field of vision; he's a great help at night times when it's dark; as I can hardly see anything and have to put my total trust in him.

It was very interesting listening to Angela explaining why she had me and it made me understand how important my role in life was.

I began to enjoy living with Angela at her house in Mincers Close, Lordswood, as we went out to different places and did different things. One day, Angela said, 'right Timber, we're going somewhere special. When we get there you are to behave yourself.' Right I thought. On went the harness and I immediately knew I was meant to work. We left the house to catch a bus. We eventually arrived at a house in Gillingham to visit Angela's friend Jackie. Jackie opened the door and to my surprise there was a playmate for me! Now, I want you to use your imagination, here's me quite tall and there's this very small dog which was a Yorkie, who could virtually stand underneath me. It was a dwarf! There I was looking down at this Yorkie who thought she could scare me by barking. We were taken into Jackie's dining room and the patio doors were open. Then I heard Angela saying 'is it alright to take Timber off his lead?' When Jackie said yes, she unclipped me and I ran outside and nearly went head first into a big pond! It was full off something I couldn't work out and my nose was inching towards the water then Jackie's voice shouted out 'no Timber, leave'. I thought, oh well, then went running around the garden with the Yorkie dog. When Angela and Jackie weren't looking, my curiosity was getting the better of me so I went back to the pond and looked down. I could see this thing and it was staring right up at me. I got closer still to the water, got my tongue out to have a lick and all of a sudden I heard Jackie shout out 'NO Timber'. My head shot up wondering what the fuss was about. I later found out that the things in the water were called fish. I still can't work out what's so special about them; they just looked like fun and something different to play with.

Angela and I did have some lovely bonding time together. There was a game I used to play which I worked out all by myself. If I carried my ball upstairs and lay down on the landing facing the stairs, I could to put my ball on the top step and then nudge it with my nose and it would bounce all the way downstairs. I would then run after it. It was such fun! Angela would stand there laughing at me.

The activity that we did together which I absolutely loved to bits was called grooming. It was heaven. Angela would fetch out my comb and brush and a towel for me to lay on. She'd call me over and get me to sit or stand and then ran her fingers all the way through my fur backwards loosening any fur that needed to come out. This used to make me all wobbly in the knees and I would have difficulty in standing up. I just wanted to lie down, roll on my back and stretch my legs out and signal for her to comb my tummy. I did have a particular worry though; this was when she was grooming me with the metal tooth comb. You see, my willy is very delicate and I cringed when she went near it with that thing. There have been a few close encounters and I gave a sigh of relief when she managed to miss it. Only men can imagine and understand what it would do to you and bring tears to your eyes. When Angela grooms me, it brings us closer and there have been times when I have started licking her, well she needs grooming too!

Who says dog's don't have expensive tastes? I do. Angela was sitting on the sofa one day counting out her money to pay the rent on the house where we were living and I noticed a £20 note had fallen onto the floor. Angela recounted the money and couldn't understand why she was £20 short when everything had been correct a moment ago. She got up to look for the missing £20 note. I was just lying there being quiet, and I had seen it and wasn't going to tell her where it was. I waited till Angela went out of the room and then went to pick it up. I took it over to my bed and started to have a good chew on it, but she came downstairs and looked at me and said 'what have you got there? I tried hiding it and acted as if I didn't have anything but I discovered that she was smarter than me. She came over and opened my mouth and extracted one wet, soggy £20 note!

A few months after that incident, Angela got a telephone call from her daughter Clair. All I got was one side of the conversation so didn't have any idea of what it was all about. All I heard was 'that's lovely, I would love to do that'. Do what? I wondered. It was about a week after the call when I noticed that Angela was feeling excited.

She got me all groomed and shiny, took me outside so that I could do my business and then placed the harness on me. We went out of the door and instead of going the usual way, she commanded me to turn left. We crossed several roads and I thought, we're going to Clair's, then all of a sudden as we were getting closer to a school that I knew her grandson attended, she commanded me to 'find right' and turn into the school yard. We walked up the school path towards the office where Clair was waiting for us.

Clair led Angela and me into a hall. Angela sat down on a chair and then told me to sit. We were waiting there when suddenly the doors were opened and a large group of children came filing into the hall and sat down on the floor in rows in front of us.

I soon found out what this was about. It was a talk about summer attire, about summer clothes and sunglasses. Sunglasses of course are very important to shade your eyes from the glaring sun and protect them from damage. The school was raising money for good causes and Guide Dogs were one of the charities that they were supporting. Angela stood up and gave a talk about why she had me and what we did together; teaching children that there are people who cannot see or have difficulties seeing. After the talk, the children were allowed to ask questions and then they came up to stroke me. I liked that.

A few of the children were picked to have their pictures taken with Angela and me; Angela's grandson being one of them. These pictures were taken by a reporter from a local newspaper. Fame again!

Angela had and still has, a special friend called Maria. She used to come and stay with us when she was going through difficulties in her personal life. On one particular weekend Maria came to stay with us and, if ever you could hear two women talking the hind leg off a donkey, it would be Maria and Angela.

They were watching a video one night. Maria was sitting on the settee and Angela was seated in the armchair. Neither of them were anywhere near the television when suddenly the brass dragonfly ornament on top of the set went flying across the room. It startled both the women and I have to admit that it startled me too. Especially when you've got this thing flying towards you and you are just lying there minding your own business. Angela spoke out to a Spirit who had come to visit us and was letting us know it was there by knocking the ornament off the television set telling it to 'pack it in and behave itself'. It all went quiet after that.

The following incident will show you how active the spirits were at Angela's house in Mincers Close. Angela went away for a week to The Arthur Findlay College near Stanstead in Essex. Maria came to stay at Angela's house a few days before she returned home. It was about two in the morning when Maria felt herself being pushed over to one side of the bed; so much so that her nose was touching the bedside cabinet. She shouted out to the Spirit in terms that left no room for misunderstanding that it should make itself scarce. She slept the rest of the night with the bedside lamp on.

It was on that same weekend whilst Angela was cooking a Sunday roast that Maria said she would take me out for a walk. We went to the local woods that were nearby and when we arrived there she unleashed me and I went off exploring. Maria was walking way behind me and I'd gone round some bushes and trees when I saw something I didn't like and felt it was dangerous for Maria to go any further. I ran back to Maria and started barking. This really worried Maria as she knew I didn't bark, in fact no one has ever heard me bark and it surprised me to use my voice. I was so anxious that Maria was not to go any further along the path. Thankfully she listened to me. She put the leash back on me and we returned home. That was a close shave.

I used to love it when Angela's family came to visit. There would be Clair and her husband Colin with their three children. There were two boys; Taylor who was the eldest, Cameron and Amelia who was the baby of the family. Everybody called her Millie. Angela also had two sons who lived close by, they were Grant and Martin.

My first Christmas with Angela was a special one. There was a big family get together, not only were Angela's children and grandchildren there, there were other members of the family too. Angela's eldest brother David turned up with his wife Jo, along with her sister Belinda with her husband James and their children Samantha and Tim. It was a full house! I was made such a fuss of as it was the first time I had been introduced to everyone. I did get tired after a while and went back into my bed to sleep off the festivities.

We celebrated the New Year very quietly. Angela had made a very important decision; after three years of being separated from her husband, she was now going to file for divorce. I sensed a new determination within Angela. It was in the January of 2008 when she met a lady called Michelle who came round to see her for a reading. They got on so well that they became friends.

Angela and Michelle used to take it in turns to host each other to lunch, and this usually involved a bottle of wine. One day, when it was our turn to go to Michelle's for lunch, Angela had a couple of small glasses of wine which made her feel tipsy. When the time came to go home, Angela placed the harness on me and said 'take me home Timber'. I escorted her safely home to her door, after which she sorted me out before having a snooze on the sofa.

Every dustbin day, Angela used to take out the rubbish to the kerb at the front of the house. On this particular day, Angela went out of the front door leaving it on the latch. She not only left the front door open, she also left the living room door wide open too. I saw my opportunity to escape. I wandered across the road and then made my way along the path to the next road. I was having a whale of a time and could hear Angela's voice calling my name in the distance. I was having so much fun that I ignored her.

When she eventually found me, Angela was frantic with worry. Not only because I had escaped, but because I could have got run over. Luckily for me, we were living in a quiet residential area. I did get a severe telling off for causing such a fright, though.

I did have a special trait. Whenever we stopped anywhere, like waiting for a bus or talking to anyone, Angela would drop my harness down and I would lean against her leg. If Angela moved slightly to one side, I'd be leaning so much that I would fall in that direction.

I loved meeting people. Whenever Angela had visitors come to the house, I would attempt to go with her to greet them at the door and make a fuss of them too. Angela would command me to stay. Once the visitor had entered and sat down, Angela would then tell me to come and say hello. There were times when visitors might come to the house and I would ignore them. This was because they made me wary and as a result I didn't like them.

Angela and I were settling into a lovely routine. It was the month of April 2008 when Angela received a telephone call from her landlady that she was being given notice to quit the property where we were living. Angela was given two weeks' notice but due to legal requirements, we did not leave Mincers Close until May that year.

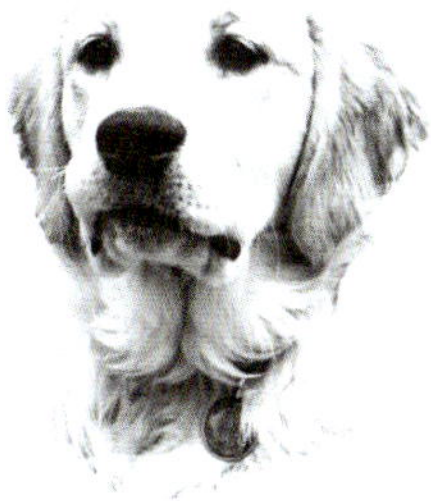

Chapter 4

Moving and our new home.

Hello again. As you can imagine, Angela and I were rather busy settling into our new home. I've had to wait several weeks before getting up onto the chair to work the computer as Angela had to get a company to install the internet connection and put the computer together. This allowed me to have a rest, as this writing lark is hard work.

Now, where were we? Ah yes, the move.

On the morning of the move, Angela called me upstairs to come and see her and she did a rare thing. She tapped the bed and gave me permission to get up onto it and lay beside her. I didn't need asking twice! I was up on the bed like a shot and snuggled down beside her. She was talking to me saying that we were moving today and it was a new beginning. The weather outside was very sunny and bright at seven in the morning. She told me that I would be going to stay with Clair whilst everything was being moved out of the house.

I stayed at Clair's until it was time for me to be taken to my new home. I must admit I was a little anxious wondering if it was going to be the same lady and not another family I was being taken to.

Clair got me into the back of the car and we started our journey. I was looking out of the window and thinking to myself, where am I going? Eventually after about half an hour Clair pulled up outside a house in Twydall Lane, Gillingham. She let me out of the car and we walked up a gravel drive to the front door. Clair rang the doorbell. Angela answered the door to let us into the house. She was very pleased to see me.

It turned out that the house had been divided into two flats and Angela had the ground floor. As you entered the flat, there was a small hall. Off the hall to the immediate right was the utility room while ahead to the right was Angela's bedroom. Ahead to the left of the front door was the living room and to the left of the hall was the bathroom.

We went through the living room to the massive kitchen/diner. There were boxes everywhere still waiting to be unpacked but I was happy to see that my bed, bowls and toys were there waiting for me.

Angela and I soon settled down. She let me sleep in her bedroom as it was a strange place and she kept talking to me telling me that we were going to be alright living in the new flat. It took nearly a week before everything was sorted and we were back into a routine again.

Angela was exploring the area. She was looking for somewhere to take me for my runs and free time. The funny thing was, she had lived in Twydall many years before, and it was like coming full circle. Not long after we'd moved, Angela decided she wanted to go out and catch a bus to take me to a park that was quite a way from home. Angela commanded me to go to the kerb. It was a totally new area for me and I had to learn a new route. Angela then stood back and pointed right and told me to go in that direction. We walked up a long road and I could hear a lot of traffic up ahead and realised we were approaching a very busy main road. Angela then told me to find right and we turned and walked along the road until we reached a side street called Eastcourt Lane. She made me sit again and then gave the command to find the bus stop. I took her straight to it.

We'd been waiting there for quite a while when another lady came to the bus stop. Angela asked her if she knew when the next bus was due. They then got talking as Angela blurted out that she was new to the area having only just moved there and that she was a 'Spiritualist Medium'. Angela did say later that she wondered why she had told the woman she was a Medium. Anyway, the bus came and the lady introduced herself as Tracey. We all sat down at the same seat, me being placed between Angela's legs to keep me out of the way of anyone else and to stop them tripping over me.

Tracey asked Angela what my name was to which she replied 'Timber'. Tracey was thrilled to bits at this as she used to have a dog, who had since passed, who was called Timber. Tracey believed that we are meant to meet people for a reason. They exchanged telephone numbers and Angela gave Tracey our address as she had asked if it would be alright to come round to show Angela a picture of her dog, Timber.

We only had a short ride before getting off and walking down a road to find a big park. I had a whale of a time, sniffing around everywhere, discovering new things and trying to make new friends; doggie friends that is. After a while Angela called me to come back to her, and for once I was a good boy. I was really enjoying myself in this new park.

Tracey later came to our house in Twydall Lane and showed Angela her dog's picture and they had such a lot in common that they became good friends. Tracey used to come round to the flat quite a lot and she and Angela used to talk about Spiritual stuff. It was on one such occasion that Angela asked Tracey if she happened to know of a Medium as she wanted something called a reading. I didn't know what this was. I thought a reading was to do with reading a book.

Tracey said she knew of a guy called Kevin who didn't live far away. Angela rang him to make an appointment and went to see him that very same evening. Kevin was to play a very important part in Angela's life.

I will mention that Tracey became a firm friend of mine. I was very picky about my food. I was given dried food once a day in the evenings along with my water. I just got bored with it and said 'nope, not eating it'. This got Angela worried that I might be going down with an illness. She would leave the food in my bowl for a couple of hours and then as instructed by Guide Dogs, had to throw it away. Angela took me to the vet's to make sure that I was well and I was given the all clear. She then rang Guide Dogs for some advice and they told her to keep putting the food down for me each evening and that I would eventually eat it. They were right.

It was on one particular evening when Tracey came round to the flat for a girlie chat and a drink that Angela mentioned about me not eating well. Tracey asked her what I was having and when she heard that it was dried food every day, she was mortified! Angela mentioned that she had a piece of steak in the fridge and Tracey proceeded to cook it, chop it up and plonked it in my bowl. Needless to say I was there in seconds and the bowl was going around the kitchen with me trying to lick every piece of meat and juice out of it. I never got steak again after that. The reason why I have my dried food is that it's carefully weighed so that I don't put on weight. If I did, then the harness would not fit me and then Angela would not be able to go out with confidence without me being there. It will also cause me other health issues. It was for my own good and Angela's, so it seems.

We were now in June 2008. Life seemed to be getting busier. We were going out more and more to different places and meeting new people. Angela discovered more information about the KAB. They had a social gathering once a month when they visited different places. A mini bus would come and pick us up from a car park in Chatham and take us to wherever they had decided to go that day. We went Ten Pin Bowling but the venue was a very noisy place. I didn't like it very much. Another place was a vineyard where we were shown how the cider and wine were made followed by lunch. Goodneston Park was a lovely place, very peaceful and again a café which served lovely smelling lunches. The Walpole Bay Hotel in Cliftonville was Angela's favourite place. It was very oldie worldy. One thing I'd noticed was that every trip involved a pit stop at a café to have a cup of tea. Most of the people on the bus were elderly and Angela was the youngest of them all. I enjoyed those days out. The destinations were exciting but the travelling got a bit boring after a while.

Most of the time I enjoyed going out with Angela. She became very relaxed and we worked well together. There were some problems though. Not I hasten to add with Angela, but with the people around us. This used to cause Angela a lot of frustration and at times anger which reduced her to tears.

We were walking around in Boots in the Pentagon Shopping Centre, Chatham. Angela stopped to look at something and I was sitting there minding my own business when all of a sudden a small child came running up to me. I thought, oh goody, someone to make a fuss of me. Just imagine the shock when this little boy promptly smacked me on the nose hard and ran away. The mother saw what had happened and didn't even apologise for her son's behaviour. She just pulled him away and said in a laughing voice 'no, you mustn't do that, mummy will buy you some sweets'. My nose did hurt and Angela stroked me to comfort me. We also had problems with the elderly. There's nothing wrong with them except that they think they can get away with anything with regards to guide dogs. Many a time Angela would be trying to do her shopping or go somewhere and we would be going our merry way when all of a sudden a person might stop us in our tracks and want to stroke me. Angela at times would have to refuse because it states clearly on my harness, 'please don't distract me I'm working'. But they always came out with the comment, 'I know I shouldn't, but I will'. There have been times when Angela has refused to let a person stroke me. They would then become rude and say something like 'I donate to Guide Dogs you know'. That doesn't make any difference. If only people would realise how distressing it can be for Angela or indeed any person who has a guide dog to be treated in this way.

Angela's friend Kevin came round to the flat one day and I was introduced to him. I really liked him. I could hear Angela and Kevin talking quite a lot, mostly about Spiritual stuff. When they started going on about that, I would go back into my bed and let them get on with it. Kevin was even more of a special friend to me. When Angela and he were talking and were having a cup of tea, they had biscuits. Now, when the biscuit barrel was opened my head would shoot up as I knew what was in there. I would then very slowly get out of my bed, keeping my head down below the table as I knew Angela couldn't see me, and Kevin would hand me a biscuit. There were times when Angela just happened to look down and she could see the top of my head and I would get this 'Timber, back into your bed'. And Kevin would get a telling off for giving me a biscuit!

It wasn't just Kevin that was coming to the house. Once a week Angela was having people round on a Tuesday evening. They would all come in and greet one another then sit down at the kitchen table. All of a sudden it would go quiet and I would hear Angela saying that she would be opening the 'circle' in prayer. 'Circle? What's going on here I'd ask myself?' Once the prayer had been said I noticed how calm the room became, then I'd notice that we had extra visitors in the room. The humans couldn't see them but I could. I'd creep out of my bed and sit next to the person that was closest to me but most of the time I went and sat beside Kevin. This feeling was lovely. I can't describe it, only that I felt very peaceful to the point that I had to lay down and sleep until it was all finished. From what I understand after listening to the people around the table, they were learning how to communicate with spirit and pass on the messages that they received. They were using different tools to make their link stronger or to find the way that was best for them to work. They also sent out healing to each other and then out to their family and friends and they would also send healing out to the world, not forgetting the animal kingdom. I liked the sound of that. After that, there was nibbles and tea; it was a lovely get together of likeminded people.

Angela also had people visit her who wanted readings, guidance, healing or just a shoulder to cry on. She really enjoyed her work as well as visiting Spiritualist Churches and centres. Mind you, she didn't have many bookings for this kind of work at that time.

Whilst all of this was going on, having decided on New Year's Eve of 2007 that she was going to start divorce proceedings from her second husband, Angela's divorce was finalized in September 2008. She was a free woman once again. Her life was going to change altogether; for the better I hasten to add.

Oh! I forgot to mention about another member of the family joining us. It was whilst I was having a little break from typing that I saw the picture which reminded me.

Tracey came round one day and happened to mention that her cat had just given birth to kittens and that she was looking for a home for them. She persuaded Angela to have a pure white kitten, but Angela wasn't really sure that the Landlord would allow it. The Landlord lived in London and would come down at odd weekends and sometimes during the week and stay in the upstairs flat. Tracey said we could train the kitten to be an indoor cat and Angela relented. Clair was also excited too as she took Angela out to buy all the things that it would need. This was when Ice entered our lives.

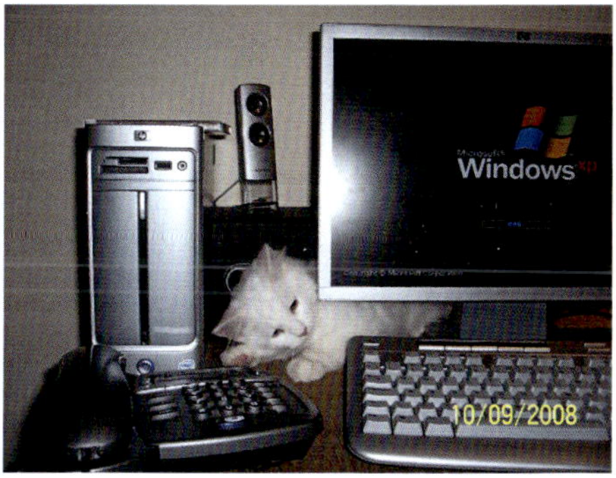

Peek-a-boo

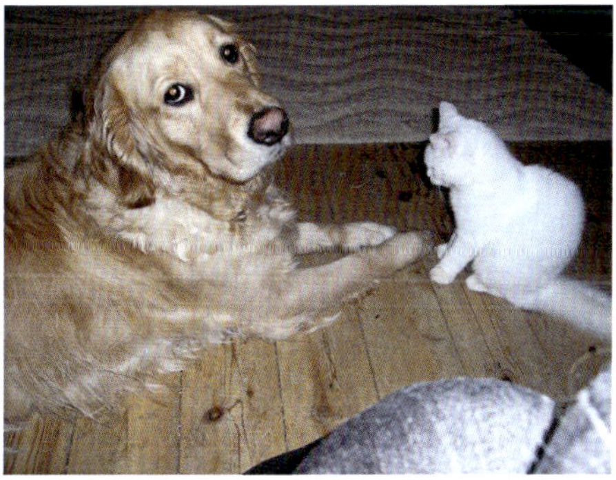

Mum, what have you done to me?

Ice was carried into the room by Tracey and placed in Angela's hand. It was a bundle of fur; not just a bundle of fur but, TROUBLE! When Ice saw me, he hissed and arched his back as if to say 'get away from me'. I just ignored him and went back to my bed. Angela didn't make a fuss of us, she just let us get on with it as she knew Ice and I would eventually get to know each other.

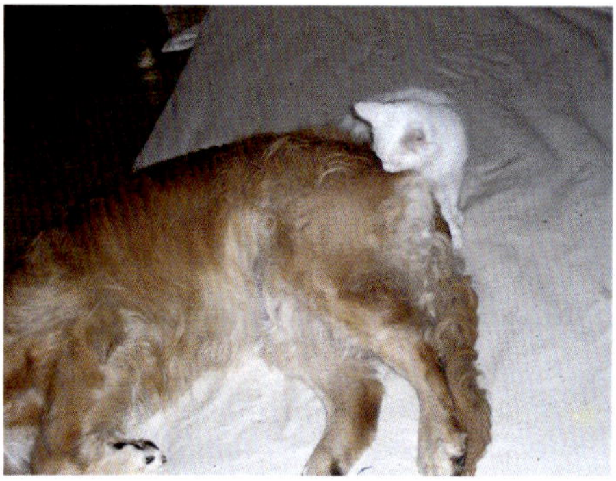

Hey, wake up!

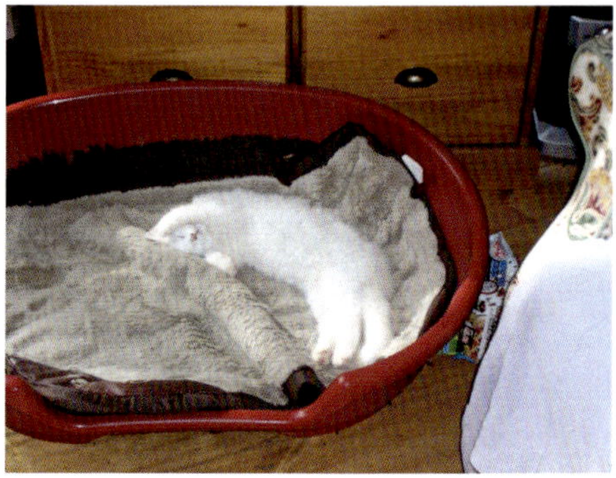

Ice taking over my bed

Oh boy! That cat just ran everywhere. He found places he shouldn't go into, like the back of the television unit, on top of the desk and behind the computer, or behind the settees (there was three of them). He tried eating MY food and drinking MY water. He also slept in MY bed which meant that I had to find somewhere else to sleep. He climbed all over me once he got used to me being there and realised that I wasn't going anywhere. He was a devil cat. He must have been as he had one blue eye and one red eye.

Then after a few weeks, he was gone.

Angela was feeling anxious about having Ice in the flat because of the Landlord. She managed to get permission for me to live there as her guide dog, but Ice, that was a different matter. Angela asked her daughter Clair if she would be able to take Ice on as she already had three cats of her own. She did take him in and he more or less ruled the roost at Clair's house too. Sadly Ice was killed in August of 2010 when he ran out in front of a passing car. It was on the same day that Angela's eldest son Grant got married.

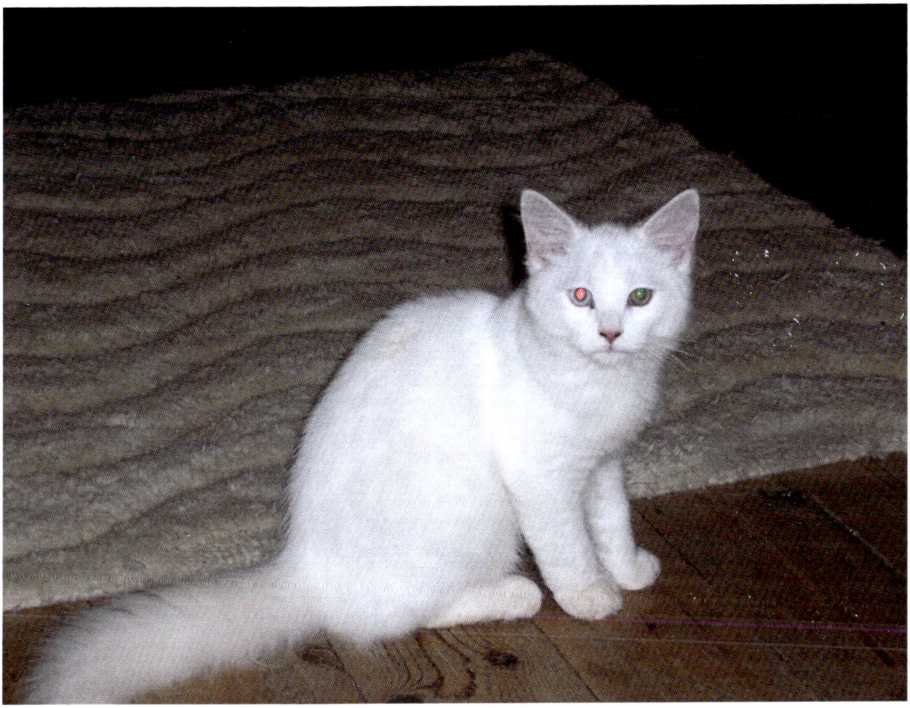

In Memory of Ice 2008 - 2010
(Did you notice one red eye and one blue eye?)

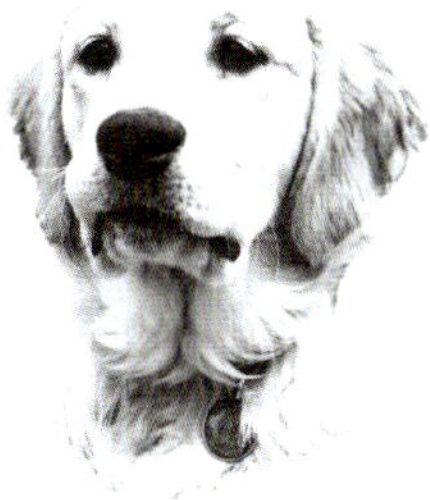

Chapter 5

A New Man Coming Into Our Lives

One day, Angela woke up early; she seemed unsettled and remained so all day. This state of affairs continued for a few weeks. I couldn't work out what was going on with her as it was rubbing off on me and I really wished that she would sort herself out!

I soon found out what it was all about. It was about eight thirty in the morning when she picked up her mobile 'phone. She dialled a number and someone answered on the other end. I do hate it when I only get one side of the conversation! Angela spoke and said 'Hello David, I don't know if you remember me, it's Angela'. Pause whilst he spoke; Angela 'I was just phoning to give you my condolences as I'd heard Val had passed away'; pause again whilst he spoke; Angela 'if you need anything or someone to talk to, please don't hesitate to contact me'; pause; Angela 'hope to see you sometime soon', then she hung up. What was all that about?!

After a little while, she appeared to be showing signs of madness. Angela began to talk to herself or should I say to someone up at the ceiling, I looked up there and couldn't see anyone and thought 'oh well'. She was muttering 'look, I've done what you told me to do' then she suddenly shouted 'okay, okay I will invite him to dinner, just get off my back'. She then started to do this texting thing. (I would never be able to do this considering the size of my paws; working on the computer is difficult enough.) When a reply came back, she had a massive smile on her face.

Later that day I found out the whole story. You humans do make it difficult for yourselves. Kevin popped round for a cuppa, (oh goody, a biscuit), and Angela explained to Kevin what had been going on. Apparently she was asleep in bed and not long before she woke up she kept hearing a voice in her ear saying 'ring David Brigenshaw'. She ignored it as she told Kevin that David had upset her many years ago and she didn't want to see him or speak to him again. But the voice kept going on and on until she relented. David's side of the conversation was yes, he remembered her very well and would love to come round for dinner.

It was a Saturday at the beginning of October2008 and Angela was feeling excited. We both went out to the shops to buy the food for the meal that evening. Angela got ready and then we waited. At about seven in the evening there was a ring at the doorbell. Angela made a last check to see if everything was ready and then went to answer the door.

I could hear voices of welcome at the door, but I was told to stay in my bed so couldn't go and see who it was. Eventually Angela and (I was soon to find out) David entered the room. They were talking quite a lot and he had a bottle of wine in his hand. When I saw the wine, I thought 'oh no, not wine, she goes all silly when she has a glass'.

Angela and David kept talking all through the evening. David was telling her how his late wife had passed. Sadly Val passed with a brain tumour within a year of her condition being diagnosed. She was a lovely lady and was well known to many people within and outside the spiritualist movement.

Then I heard Angela ask David a question. 'Why were you rude to me when I phoned you that time?' David replied 'I fell in love with you when I first saw you in 1994 and when we met again on the Isle of Sheppey after having done private readings to raise money for the Spiritualist Church there, we went back to your shop and were talking in the back room. I so very nearly broke my marriage vow to Val and you would have been the only woman that I would have done that for. I couldn't do that, so the only way to stop that happening was to cut all ties with you. I do apologise if I appeared rude, but now you know why'.

Angela replied by saying 'I didn't have a clue and I admire you for what you did'. The rest of the evening went off without a hitch and then he went home.

That was the beginning of a beautiful relationship.

Angela and David used to take it in turns to visit each other's homes at the weekends. David got home quite late in the evenings after leaving work, arriving home at about six thirty. By the time he had washed and changed, there wasn't much time for the courting during the week, so they decided to leave it to the weekends. What I haven't told you is that David is also a working Medium. He'd get home even later after he'd finished serving a church or centre during the week. Sometimes he wouldn't get home until ten thirty or eleven thirty in the evening and he would be up again at five thirty in the morning to get ready to catch the train to his job in London.

I loved it when we went to David's house. He had a big garden for me to run around in for a start. The only thing I didn't like was the stairs. They were very steep as David lived in a Victorian cottage off Nelson Road in Gillingham. Angela was gaining more and more confidence working with me even at night. It got to the point when all Angela had to say was 'we're going to David's today'. I knew how to get there and what house it was even in the dark as I knew Angela would have difficulties in seeing the numbers on the door.

I really liked David. He made Angela happy and she was smiling and laughing a lot more than she used to. We also went out more together, just the three of us.

It was in the same October when Angela had a visit from her Landlord. He was saying that he wanted to change Estate Agents and was asking Angela to move out of the flat and then move back in again. Angela was put in a very difficult position as she feared that she would lose her home if she refused. She became so upset and was crying a lot. She would have to pack up all her belongings but didn't have anywhere that they could be stored. The Landlord said that he would help her in that direction, but he never did.

The day of the 'move' came. David was there to help Angela along with some of her friends. They packed everything into a van and it was left parked down the road overnight. Angela didn't have anywhere to go as she needed to be there early in the morning to let the Agents in so she slept on a sofa which was already in the flat when she first moved in. The Agent was a condescending man who was quite rude to her but, after a short while of looking around the flat, he left.

Then it was all action stations again to get the stuff back in and unpacked. Later in the evening the Landlord came by. He asked Angela how things had gone, at which she broke down and said that it was so stressful and had cost her a lot of money to do this 'favour' for him. Not only that, the Landlord now demanded a deposit there and then whilst they were signing the new contract. Luckily Kevin was there to help out as he lent her the money. Angela vowed never again would she ever do a favour for any Landlord.

After all that excitement, life soon returned to normal. We had a lovely Christmas in Angela's flat. All of the family came round. Angela's sister Belinda, brother in-law James and their children visited on Christmas Day. Then, on Boxing Day, her daughter Clair and her family called round. David wasn't with us over this Christmas as, before he had got together with Angela, he had promised to spend the holiday with his brother Richard and his family in Essex. They missed each other terribly as Angela was all alone on Christmas morning.

New Year came bringing a feeling of new things to come. We were still having people coming round to Angela's circle. By this time, they were working with crystals, tarot cards, sand, paper and the one thing I liked best, healing; I couldn't get enough of it. It was on 11 February 2009, before everyone arrived for the circle, that David arrived earlier than usual. He seemed a little nervous somehow. Angela was chatting away, asking him if he would like a cup of coffee. Instead of replying 'yes, please' he said 'Angela, come over here a minute'. Angela was a little puzzled and a bit apprehensive thinking that there was something seriously wrong. He then got Angela to sit on his lap and said 'will you marry me?' whilst fumbling around in his trouser pocket to bring out a little box which he handed to her. Angela didn't hesitate and said 'yes!' She opened the box and placed the engagement ring on her finger. There was a lovely celebration after the circle meeting that evening. Everyone congratulated them both.

Maria still came round to stay with us from time to time and she used to bring a friend with her called Wendy. Wendy was a very troubled lady and deeply depressed. Angela and Maria used to try and cheer her up by having girlie nights indoors. On one particular occasion the weather took a turn for the worse, it snowed! Yippee, I thought. Mind you, you didn't get much chance to roll around it in our little scrap of a back garden. We did go out to the front garden which was much bigger and I was in my element. Angela took me round to the nearby big park that we went to regularly and

I had the time of my life. Shame I couldn't do the angel wings in the snow, can you just imagine it?

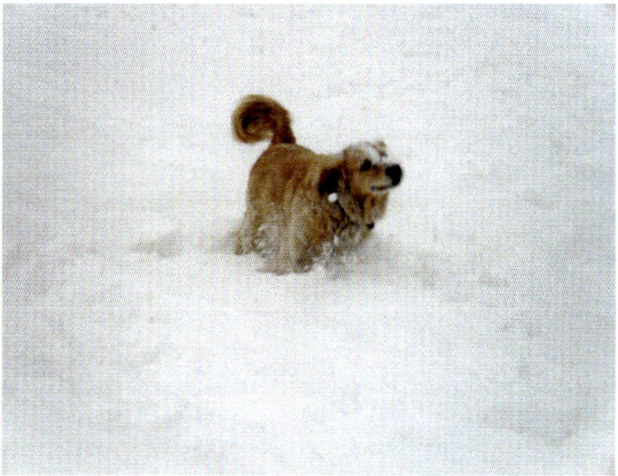

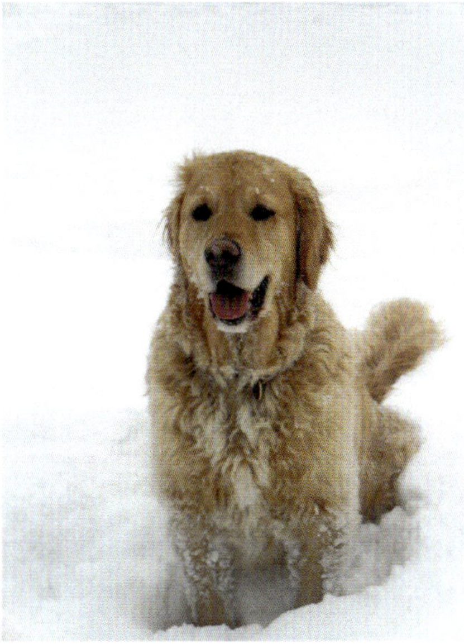

In it up to my elbows. (above)
Loving snow! (right)

It was about this time that Mel came into our lives.

Wendy had a friend that she had known for years and said that she, Mel, would love to meet Angela and Maria. They made arrangements to meet at The Cricketers pub in Rainham for lunch. We all met up and I took to Mel straight away; she was nice. I was lying under the table listening to everything that was going on and when it was nearing time to go home, the girls suggested that as Mel lived just round the corner from Angela she should give us a lift home. Then I heard 'you don't need to worry about Mel's driving, she is good at it'. We all said our goodbyes and Angela and I went to Mel's car. Angela then explained that I had to sit between her legs in the front foot-well of the car. Mel was quite amused at having a dog sitting in the front and facing backwards!

They were happily chatting away whilst Mel was driving along the road when all of a sudden she had to slam her brakes on hard as there was a pedestrian on a zebra crossing. Mel was mortified! She said she would never be able to live that down having only just had people telling Angela that she was a safe driver!

One day not long after meeting Mel, Kevin was round at our flat having a cuppa when there was a ring on the doorbell. Angela wasn't expecting anyone so she answered the door and it was Mel standing there, full of apologies for coming unannounced. Angela said not to worry about it and that she was welcome to pop round any time she liked.

Mel and Kevin hit it off straight away. By the time Angela had come back into the room, I'd sneaked up to Kevin and was having my head stroked. She then told me to go and lay in my bed. I sulked my way back to bed and lay down with a hump. After about ten minutes, Angela called me over to introduce me to Mel and I was allowed to stay by her side. She was a lovely lady. There was something very special about Mel, and I could sense it.

Mel was very interested in Spiritualism. She had the gift of mediumship but didn't know how to use it or where to go to learn to develop it. Angela and Kevin said that they would help her develop her psychic skills and asked her if she would like to join the circle, which she did. To watch Mel develop was like watching a flower unfolding; she blossomed. Unfortunately, Mel was going through a lot of health and family issues of her own; she had a lot to deal with.

The situation wasn't helped when Angela received a phone call from Maria. All I could hear was shock and sorrow. When Angela finished talking to Maria, Angela called me over and started to cuddle and stroke me and said 'it's so sad', I said to her with my expressive eyes 'what's going on?' I soon cottoned on to why she was upset. Angela then got up and walked over to the telephone and dialled David's number. I heard her say 'hello darling, do you remember meeting Wendy?' He obviously said yes then she continued 'well, she committed suicide today by hanging herself.'

Maria, Mel and Angela went to the funeral the following month. Even that didn't go according to plan. On the day of the funeral, Mel came and collected Angela and then picked Maria up from the Isle of Sheppey. They all turned up at Bobbing Crematorium near Sittingbourne, parked the car and waited for others to arrive. They'd been waiting for some time and there was no sign of anyone. Mel went to the office to find out if the funeral was being held that day and when Mel came back she told them that it was the following week. Angela just burst out laughing and said 'trust Wendy.' They did eventually get to the funeral on the right day!

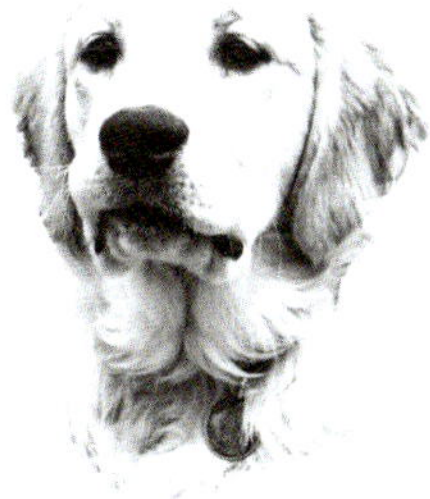

Chapter 6

Mud Glorious Mud!

The winter of 2008-09 seemed to go on forever. The snow lasted for about two weeks and it was very icy and slippery when the snow compacted. I overheard Angela talking to David about buying me snow boots. Can you imagine me walking around with four boots strapped to my feet? I just wouldn't know what to do with them. Oh bless her, she knew it was difficult for me to walk about in the snow.

When the weather warmed up during the spring of 2009, Clair phoned her mum Angela and asked if she fancied going out with her and the grandchildren to a country park, taking me of course. We went to one such place called Shorne Country Park. Was I in for a surprise!

When we arrived at the country park, Angela unleashed me and said 'go on boy'. I didn't need to be told twice, I was off. My good old nose was on overdrive with all these new smells, I didn't know where to start. Then I spotted a puddle, a very muddy puddle I hasten to add and headed straight for it. Clair and Angela shouted out 'no Timber'. Too late! Splash, and I was down in the puddle, rolling all over and coming up with a huge smile on my face; heaven. I was coated in mud. You should have heard the commotion I caused, they just laughed and said 'oh Timber, how are we going to clean you up?'

We continued to walk around the park and came across a special pond for dogs to go and jump in. Angela said 'go on Timber, in you go'. Nope, I thought, I'm not going in there! There were several other dogs all playing around and jumping into the pond. Angela and Clair said again 'go on Timber, you can if you want', nope not going in. Then I heard Angela saying 'oh well, let's go then'. That was it, I ran for the pond and was in, splash. Wow wasn't it fun, they couldn't get me back out again. When I finally decided I'd had enough I came out and then Angela, Clair and the grandchildren all ran away from me because I was going to shake myself off. They didn't want to get covered in all that muddy water.

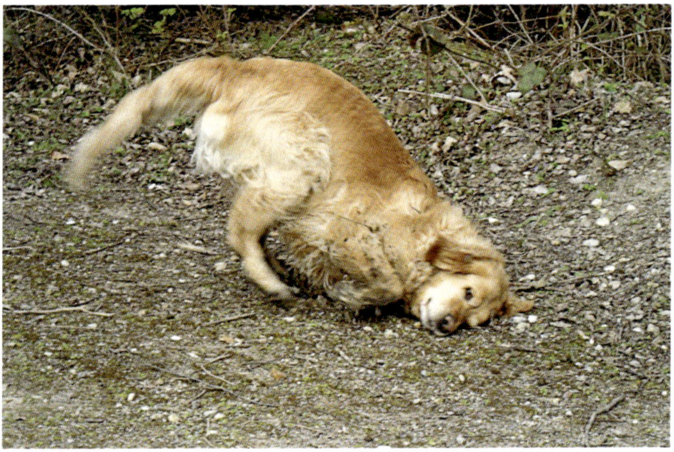

Ahh, lovely.

We all got back to the car and discovered a problem, they only had a hand towel. I needed a bath sheet. I was soaking wet. Angela and Clair dried me off as best they could then got me into the back of the car well away from them. We got home and then I was going to have more fun. Angela said 'right you, we can't have you looking like that'. She took me into the bathroom. I wondered what this was all about as I wasn't normally allowed in there. Across the bathroom was a big shower and she tried to coax me into it. But I was not going to have any of that! She then went and got the lead, clipped it on me and then she got into the shower and pulled me in, closing the door behind her. I was thinking 'now what?' She got hold of the shower head and turned on the water to start showering. I smelt like the perfume counter at Boots when I came out of there I can tell you. I'd been shampooed and conditioned to within an inch of my life!

It was also around this time that I was introduced to another doggie friend. Angela knew a lady called Sue who had got herself a Yorkie puppy. The pup was refusing to walk. Sue hit on an idea for getting her little dog Rolo to walk. She came round to our flat and introduced Rolo to me. Rolo kept barking at me which, I suppose, was her way of saying hello. The next thing I knew I was being harnessed up and we all went out for a walk. I was wondering why Sue and Rolo were walking behind me. Then I heard Sue say to Rolo, 'come on Rolo, follow Timber', which she did after several failed attempts. I can honestly say I was the one who got Rolo walking.

The one thing about Rolo was that she was always jumping over me, barking, and running around. This could get a bit wearing so I would just place my paw on Rolo and pin her to the ground as if to say 'pack it in, I've had enough'. She always quietened down after that.

There was one especially funny incident involving Rolo. Sue phoned Angela not long after we were introduced and asked her if she would like to go to the Riverside Country Park for a walk. We arrived at the park and Angela wouldn't let me off the lead for a while until we got to a certain point in the park when I was allowed to go wandering. Now, this park runs alongside the river Medway and the tide was on the ebb. When it goes out the foreshore becomes very muddy. You guessed it! I went to make a run for it and I got this very loud command 'NO, TIMBER, STOP'. Amazingly I did stop and stood where I was, but unfortunately Rolo didn't stop. She went straight in and the mud went right up to her underbelly. Sue pulled her out and she absolutely stank. Not Sue, Rolo! It took quite a few baths before the smell went away. It would have been terrible if I'd gone in and I can say this was a rare occasion when I actually listened, and was glad that I'd done so.

One of the other favourite places to go diving into the water was the sea. Clair use to pick us up and take us to Whitstable on the North Kent coast. The weather was lovely and sunny and we walked down onto the beach. It was rather pebbly and hurt my feet a little bit. We got down to the sandy bit closer to the water's edge and it was a lot more comfortable. I looked up at Angela as if to say 'can I go in, mum?' She read my eyes and unleashed me and off I went. I loved the sea, although I do remember once that I tried drinking the water and immediately started retching. It was disgusting.

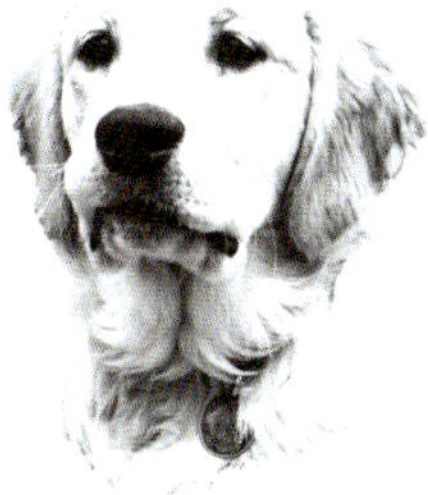

Chapter 7

Going to Wales

Angela and David had been together for nearly a year, taking turns to visit each other at weekends and going out on romantic dates. They took me everywhere with them when they were serving churches or spiritual centres, doing their demonstrations of mediumship. Everywhere I went I was made such a fuss of to the point that, when Angela and David went back to a church or spiritualist centre, everybody said hello to me first and only then remembered that Angela and David were standing behind me.

I always laid down beside Angela on the platform whilst she and David did their work. I noticed that the audience wasn't taking much notice of them; they were more interested in what I was up to. I would either be snoring or I'd get the fidgets and start moving around to try and get comfortable. When I'm not asleep, my eye brows are going nineteen to the dozen. I've been told that they are so expressive. There were cases when I even grumbled about how long the demonstration was taking and as I got older this got worse.

We were coming up to September 2009 and I was sensing some excitement in the air. Angela and David started talking about going away to Wales. This was going to be a special visit; Angela would meet her future in-laws for the first time.

The day finally arrived. David loaded up the hired car with all of my things, bedding, food, toys and bowls. I did think for a minute that I was going to stay with another family. Angela and David helped me to get into the back of the car and it took me a long time to settle down as I thought the journey was going to be a short one but it wasn't. It was a long time before David pulled into a layby to allow me to relieve myself. I tell you, I was glad to get out of the car to stretch my legs. I had a good sniff around and eventually decided I would spend a penny or two; anything to linger and take in all the different smells that were around me. Eventually they got me back into the car and we were off again.

Our next stop was Gloucester. Angela and David stopped to have lunch and to give me a break from being cooped up in the back of the car. After our lunch break, it was back into the car again. I then noticed that the roads weren't as straight; there was a lot of twisting and turning going on. I looked out of the windows and noticed there were a lot of green fields with sheep in them and these very high hills. I was later told they were mountains. I'd not seen mountains before, they were big.

We were on the road for nearly eight hours. I then heard David talking about this town called Aberaeron. He was saying that this was where his family came to do their shopping and meet their friends. Aberaeron was a lovely place, it's a seaside town with a small harbour. There was a square green in the middle of the town with a fence surrounding it. There were lots of different shops, the usual eating houses, book shops, grocers, gift and clothing shops. All the houses were painted a different colour. I then heard David saying 'not long now, we're nearly there'. About time I thought, I'm bored being in the back here.

The next village from Aberaeron was Aberarth which is situated in a deep valley. We turned left and crawled along a narrow road which opened out slightly as we neared the bungalow where David's parents lived and then the road surface changed to bumpy from smooth. Finally, we had arrived.

David got out of the car first and immediately let me out of the boot. I was so excited, this was a new adventure. I could smell something different here, it was the sea air. David's parents lived in a bungalow, (I'd never seen one of these before – I thought all houses had stairs). Their home was only about a hundred yards from the sea and there was a field opposite. In the distance I was told you could see the Snowdonia Mountains. Behind the bungalow were more fields and hills. In the field right behind the bungalow were cows and some sheep.

I was feeling so excited! I did get a welcome visit from another dog who lived just down the road nearer to the sea. Her name was Jazz and she was getting old. She always came over to anyone hoping for a treat; David's parents always gave one to Jazz every day and she thought she would push her luck and have a second go. No luck this time though!

The front door was opened and these two people came out to greet us. They were David's parents Eileen and Vic. We were all welcomed into their home. Eileen and Vic made a huge fuss of me as they love dogs, especially Eileen. I was let out into the garden to relieve myself and investigate my surroundings. I loved that place.

While I was outside, David was introducing Angela to his mum and dad and they got on like a house on fire. Angela fitted in very well.

We sat in the kitchen during the daytime and in the evenings we all trooped into the lounge. There was a lot of talking going on in the kitchen and laughter. I always laid down beside Angela but sometimes I could get in the way a bit as I'm not small. On my first night, Angela placed my food on the floor and I wasn't sure if I wanted to eat it so I ate a little and left it. I was still feeling unsure about what was going on. After a few days I did settle down when I realised that Angela wasn't going to leave me behind.

I was taken out for walks around the village, although it wasn't very big. When we came out of the front gate, we turned right then left and walked along past the village hall and some houses. We came round a bend down a short hill then walked past a closed down chapel. Beside the chapel was a bridge over the river Arth (the Bear River in Welsh). We stood on the bridge watching the water rushing down from the mountains out to the open sea. On the bridge you could see the backs of peoples' houses along the river bank. They were small houses, cottages really with two rooms up and two down.

We walked along a short alley between two houses and turned left towards the sea although you couldn't see it from this road. There used to be a school on the right hand side of the road, but it mysteriously burnt down after it closed and now there were two bungalows on the site.

We then retraced our steps after I'd decided I wanted to do my 'jobbies' and returned past the bridge over the river towards an old water mill on the left; it was a little bit dilapidated although there were people living in the cottage attached to the mill. Along this road you came to the River Arth again and then continued to the main road. You had to cross the main road, walk over another bridge and then cross the main road again to get back to where you wanted to go on the other side of the river. We went back down the road we had arrived at earlier in the day to return to David's parents' home.

David and Angela went out every day and took me everywhere they went. I saw sights that were amazing, there were lots and lots of mountains! Mind you there was a lot of rain too. It was a very wet week with some sun in between. There were a couple of times when Vic took me out for a walk along the cliff edge. David and Angela also took me down onto the beach. This was a little difficult because the beach was very pebbly; quite big pebbles in fact. Once you got onto firmer ground it was a lot better. I went flying off when Angela told me I could go, so much so I could hear in the distance behind me Angela shouting for me to come back. As you can guess, I was having none of it, again!

It was fascinating. There was a lot of seaweed about, (I'd never seen seaweed before), feathers and rubbish to investigate. I found a dead fish and I was just about to get my jaws round this when I heard a very stern command 'LEAVE'. My immediate thought was 'why'? The fish did pong a bit. I was then given the command to go off again and when I was going too far ahead of Angela and David, Angela would blow a special dog whistle. I did tend to ignore it but when she kept blowing it, I thought I'd better get back, as I was getting an ear ache.

I had the most wonderful week away in Wales, I was spoilt rotten where ever I went.

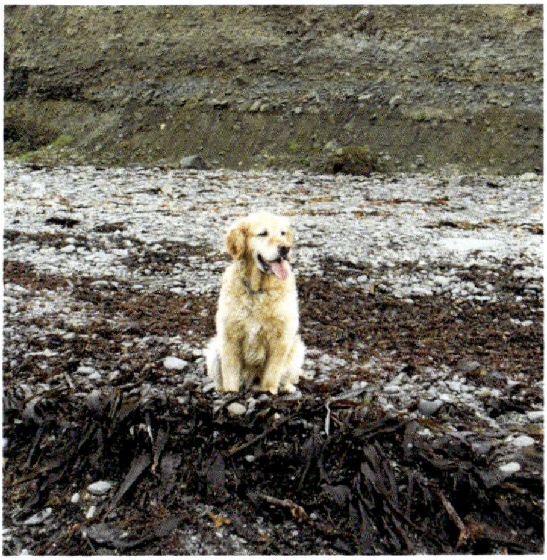

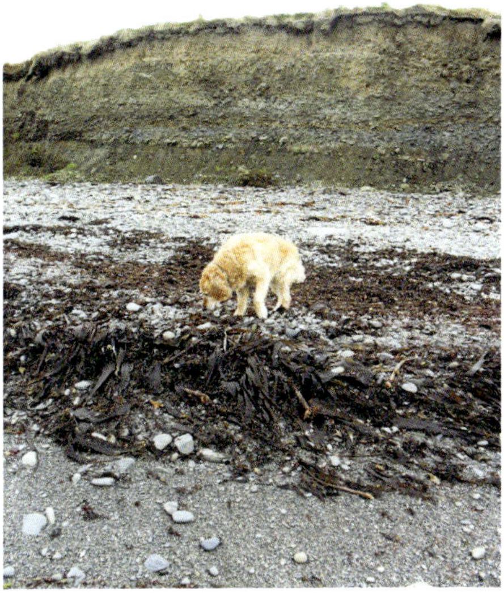

On the beach (above)
What can I find? (right)
So happy (below)

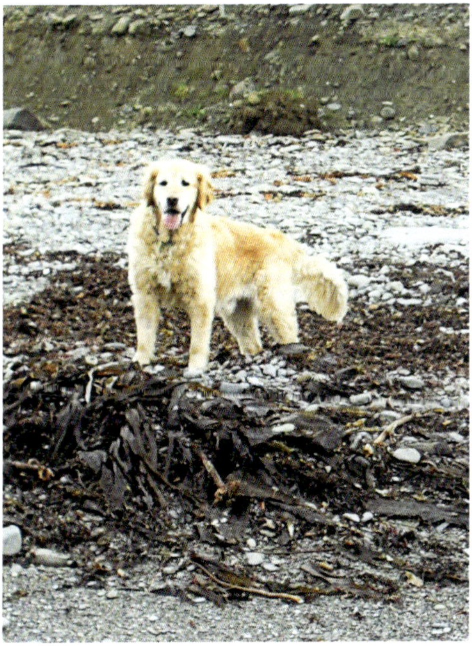

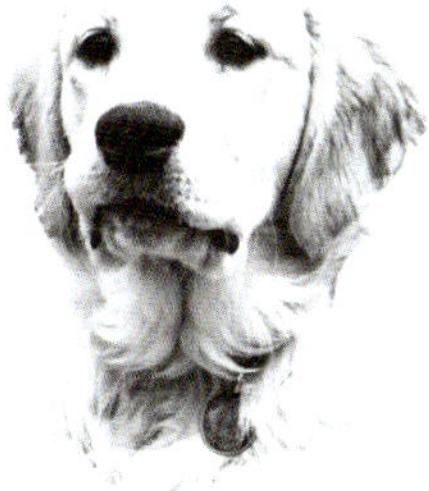

Chapter 8

Frustrating!

Angela and David had been doing a lot of work for the Spiritualist movement, including taking Divine Services around the South East of England. Before David bought a car, a lot of their journeys involved travelling by bus and then a train. Coming home late at night we had to use taxis as the buses had usually stopped running by then.

On one occasion when we emerged from Gillingham Station we crossed the High Street and began walking up the road that was opposite the station. It was a lovely warm summer's evening. I was just walking along minding my own business when all of a sudden I saw this Staffordshire terrier come running towards me. Thinking that it wanted to make friends with me I greeted him with a smile. Then, all of a sudden I was being attacked. The dog started to bite my neck and snarl at me. There was a lot of shouting going on, with everybody trying to get this dog to stop biting me around my neck. The man who owned the dog was trying desperately to get him off me. I was just sitting there a bit shocked at what was going on and

I could sense Angela and David were very angry. They shouted at the man and told him that he should have had his dog under control. The Staffy's owner wasn't very apologetic either.

When we got back to David's house, Angela checked me all over to make sure that I wasn't bleeding anywhere and kept an eye on me for the rest of the evening and the next day. I must admit, that was the first time I'd ever been attacked. I did get attacked once more on the way to a church service in Dover. There was a group of 'yobs' with cans in their hands all making a racket. We went to walk past them when all of a sudden a dog that was with them came charging out at me baring his teeth. They managed to just stop him before the dog sank its teeth into me. A lot of words were exchanged and there was a slight apology from one of the group members when they realised that I was a Guide Dog,

I didn't like working when the weather was wet. There were many times when we'd be standing on a station platform waiting for the train and the wind would be blowing a gale; wind and rain is not nice. We were on our way back home from one service and had to go and wait for a taxi at the side entrance of Gillingham Station. We turned up and asked the taxi driver if he would take us home, but he refused. He wouldn't allow us in the car even though Angela had a towel with her to place on the floor so that my wet feet wouldn't spoil the carpet. We said that under the Disability Discrimination Act the taxi driver was not allowed to refuse us unless he had an exemption to the effect that he was allergic to animals. The taxi driver got out of the car and started swearing at Angela and David. There was almost a punch-up! There had been many instances prior to this when we approached the taxi rank and the taxis would all suddenly disappear. This was the first time a taxi had refused to take us home. We did get home eventually as David phoned another taxi company he had always used in the past and they couldn't have been more helpful or friendly.

There was one train experience that particularly upset me and Angela. The train pulled into Whitstable station and a girl alighted from the train carriage in front of us. We then boarded the train and the doors shut on Angela and me. This alarmed Angela and she was quite concerned for me wondering if I'd got hurt. What had happened was that the girl who had got off the train had pressed the button to shut the doors on us for 'a joke'. Angela complained to the conductor who happened to be in the same carriage as us and he said and did nothing; amazing.

The other thing that Angela found extremely frustrating was when we were walking along a path across the playing field near to our home to get to where we needed to go. In this field there would always be dogs off their lead having a good run around. Of course I was never allowed to play in this field because I might start to associate it with fun and games and not walk across it properly as a working guide dog should.

I'd get so excited when I saw other dogs; even more so when the dogs would come up to me and totally distract me. It was worse for Angela as she might not have seen the other dog approach. I would then start going all over the place and this would totally throw her out. Her command of 'walk on' didn't work either because the other dog would not leave me alone. Angela would then have to stop completely making me sit down to wait for the other dog to be called back by its owner. Most owners would come up with the excuse that 'it's being friendly and wants to play'. Angela would then try and explain that their dog's antics were making it very difficult for her to continue with her journey. A lot of owners would then get all huffy and could be quite rude. Angela would then continue her journey feeling very angry, frustrated and sometimes reduced to tears. It was so upsetting.

Angela and I have been refused service when entering a food shop. The shop assistant told Angela that she had to leave me outside as I wasn't allowed in the shop. Angela tried to explain to the shop assistant that, as a guide dog, I was allowed entry into all shops; she even showed him the Environmental card stating this fact but the shop assistant wouldn't have any of it, she still had to leave. Angela was fuming! Angela then spoke to Guide Dogs about what had happened and they said that they would sort it out for her. It was a couple of months later when David noticed there was a sticker placed on the shop door saying Guide Dogs welcomed.

Mind you I did create some frustration for Angela myself.

As I got older, I decided that I wasn't going to like lifts. When I noticed that we were heading towards a lift I would start to back away from it. We would then have to take the stairs. Angela didn't let me get away with this though, she had a trick up her sleeve. She would have a tasty bit of ham in her bag and would get this ready to entice me into the lift. Once I got the hang of lifts again, she stopped giving me the treat. Problem solved!

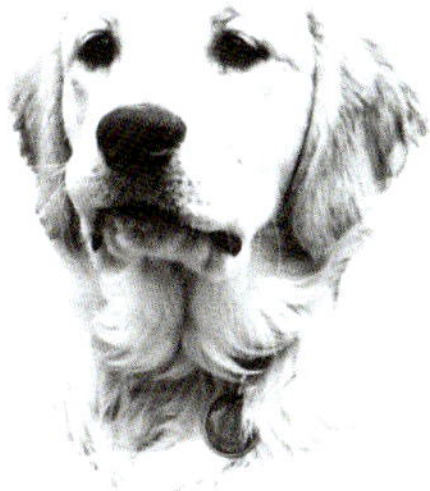

Chapter 9

Oh Boy!

As I've said, Angela's friend Mel was deeply interested in Spiritualism. She wanted to learn how to develop her psychic abilities, not only to give readings, but also to channel healing energies from Spirit. Kevin used to come round as well to help teach Mel. As you know, I liked her a lot as she was a very special lady. She had a special way with me; I was putty in her hands when she placed them on my head or body. I would then lie straight down on the floor and relax.

She also taught me to sing. (I'm sniggering here.) Yes, sing. Mel had a lovely voice and she would sing quite a lot when she was happy or Angela was playing a particular tune that Mel recognised. Mel would then start to sing to me and dance around me. I would then start to howl (singing to you and me). Angela would burst out laughing. I'm afraid to say that Angela's voice is not good but David's voice, now, that is something else. He comes from a Welsh background and was a choir boy. He has a beautiful voice.

Mel asked Angela if she and I would like to go round to visit her at her house. She said that she had a big garden for me to run around in. It was a lovely sunny day and Mel and Angela were sitting out in the garden. I was running all over the place trying to identify the different smells. This was something I missed in my own scrap of a garden.

I was quite a way up the garden in the flower border when I came across a ball. Now I like balls, especially tennis balls. I got hold of it and took it back to the lawn to pull it apart and chew it. I had a whale of a time doing this until the ball was totally destroyed.

Later that same evening I started to feel unwell. Angela and David had gone to bed and luckily for me their bedroom door was still open. I'd been sick all over the kitchen floor, and when I got into the bedroom, David could hear me retching and being sick again. Angela couldn't hear me at all as she had taken her hearing aids out. I kept being sick all night, I felt so weak.

The next morning, Angela rang the Wigmore Veterinary Surgery in Maidstone Road, Rainham. They made an appointment for me to come in straight away. David had already left for work earlier that morning so Angela phoned Kevin to ask if he would take us.

I could barely get into the car, I was so weak and shaky. I tried to curl up on the floor of the car but there wasn't much space for me to lie down. We arrived at the vet's and I was taken into the consulting room straight away where the Vet was waiting for me. He took notes and asked Angela questions. I was examined and the

Vet said to Angela that she would have to leave me behind. They wanted to keep me in because they didn't like the look of me.

Angela gave me a quick cuddle and reassured me that I would be okay. I went off with the nurse who then gave me an injection and took some blood samples. I had all sorts of things done to me; they even put a drip into me to help replace the fluids that I'd lost. Oh, I forgot to mention, I had messed everywhere, it was very runny and smelt awful. The Vet said he would ring Angela later in the day to tell her how I was and what was causing my illness.

Late in the afternoon on the same day, Angela came and picked me up again on the condition that I was to return the following day. The test results came back saying that I had Gastroenteritis.

I was laying on a sheet on the floor in the living room. I was still messing myself lying on the floor, I couldn't stop it happening. Mel came round to visit me. She was feeling guilty as it was the ball in her garden that had made me so ill. She came and knelt beside me, I looked at her and placed my paw on her and said 'I'm alright', and did that thing with my eyes that melts everyone's heart. I looked into her eyes and she started to cry. Angela told Mel that I was okay and she had nothing to be sorry for.

I went back to the vets for two more days, being monitored and put back on the drip to keep my fluids up. It took me a couple of weeks to be able to eat properly, I was being fed chicken and rice and gradually they weaned me off it and replaced it with my own food. I still didn't have enough strength to go out for long walks, so

Angela took me out for gentle strolls, not taking me far. Each day the walk would get longer and I was soon back to my bouncing self.

Whilst I was ill, Angela was asking for healing to be sent to me from her friends on Facebook. I didn't realise how popular I was.

That wasn't the only time I was unwell.

Angela and her daughter Clair had gone out for a couple of hours to buy things for Angela's wedding. It would have been difficult to take me as it involved dressing rooms. Trying to take me into a dressing room is very difficult when Angela is trying on something.

They had not long gone after making sure that I'd gone outside and done my 'spend' when I started to feel unwell. I tried very hard to not do anything but in the end I had to give in.

Angela and Clair came home. Angela came into the kitchen first and walked over towards the cooker. She then went sliding across the kitchen floor. She had stood right in my very runny poo. It was not only runny, it stank! I didn't get shouted at though. Angela knew there must have been something wrong because I didn't get out of my bed to greet her, I stayed put.

She cleared up the mess and kept an eye on me for the rest of the day. There was no repeat performance I'm glad to say. Angela did put me back on chicken and rice and rested me for a couple of days to make sure I had got over whatever it was that had upset me.

It was due to being ill the first time that I refused to walk through the Pentagon Shopping Centre in Chatham. We'd gone into town to do some shopping and Angela commanded me to 'find the Pentagon'. I took her there and we walked through the doors. I'd only gone a few yards into the Pentagon when I stopped. Angela commanded me to 'walk on'; I just refused. She tried dropping the harness down and walking me through the Pentagon on a leash. Nope, wasn't having that either, I just turned round and went back out the way we came in.

Angela tried on several occasions to get me to walk through the shopping centre and I was still doing the very same thing. Angela became worried about this so she phoned Lesley at Guide Dogs and explained what was happening with me.

Lesley came and picked us up and took us into Chatham. We walked through the High Street. Yes I was doing fine but then Lesley asked Angela to take me into the Pentagon. Again I did the same thing as before, I refused to budge. The reason I didn't walk through the shopping centre was that the floor was very shiny with silver manhole covers. This was apparently triggering a memory of me being at the vets and I didn't like it.

How did they get me out of it? Through my belly!

Lesley enticed me through the shopping centre with titbits from her pocket. I knew they were there. The first time we walked through, Angela had to hold onto Lesley so she could guide her through the shopping centre and Angela just held the lead and kept encouraging me by telling me that I was a good and wonderful boy. After several attempts, I got used to the floor and knew that there was nothing to be frightened of.

Angela breathed a sigh of relief when I started to work properly again.

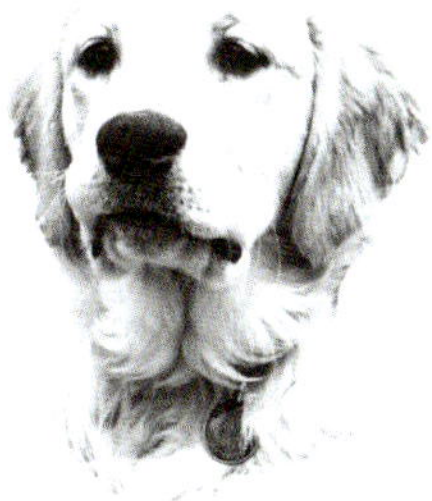

Chapter 10

The Hen Night and Angela's Wedding

It was now September 2010, the month when Angela and David were getting married. There was a lot of excitement in the air, a lot of comings and goings, talking about the wedding, the food and the guests. They even made a trial wedding cake that nearly blew your head off with the amount of alcohol in it! Not that I was allowed any.

It was the beginning of September and there was this talk of a hen do. What? Were we going to have chickens in the house? No, Angela's best friend Maria had organised a party to be held at Angela's flat. She had arranged for families and friends to come round for a pamper afternoon and into the evening followed by Chinese take away and lots and lots of booze.

There was lots of laughter and balloons. What those ladies did with those balloons boggled the doggie mind! It was fun for me up to the time when one of the balloons burst. This made us all jump and I became very frightened and decided this wasn't fun for me anymore. I started shaking all over and kept wanting Angela to cuddle me. In fact a cuddle from anyone would have been okay.

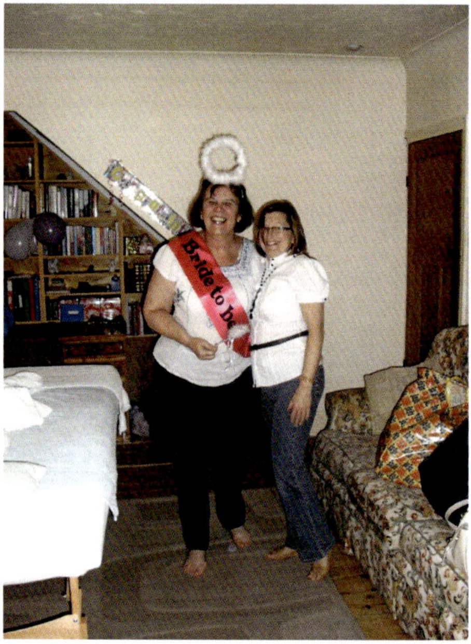

A right fairy! Angela with Maria.

As I was frightened, Angela took me into her bedroom and turned the lamp on along with the radio for company. I didn't like being left in there, I wanted to be in with the fun that was going on. But at the same time, I was frightened of the balloons. So I guessed I had to stay there.

It was the day before the wedding. Maria had come over to stay with Angela; Maria was doing all the cooking for the evening buffet. They worked together during the day cooking the food; I must say, it did smell rather good in the flat, but unfortunately I didn't get any of the goodies.

It was late afternoon when Mel arrived and I noticed that all of my things were disappearing again. First my bed and then the food and toys. I was wondering what was going on. Angela got me into Mel's car and we drove to somewhere I'd never been to before. We arrived at this house and walked up to the door and a lovely lady opened it and greeted us. Not only did the lady greet us, two other dogs were there. Playmates!

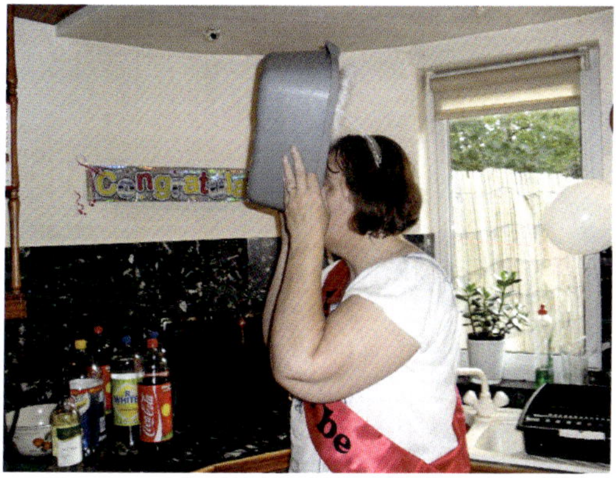

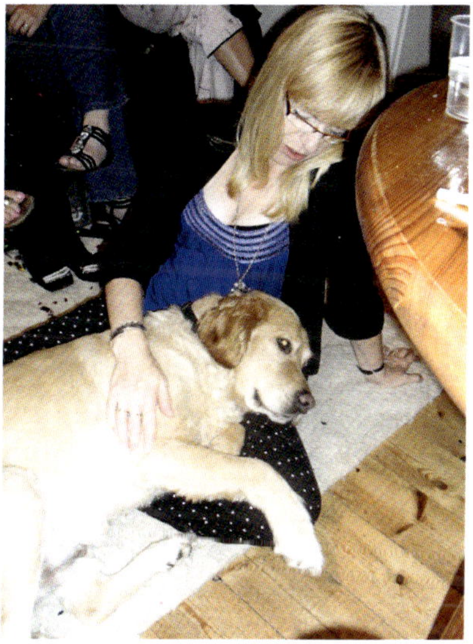

Drinking the Pimm's... (above)
Being made a fuss off by Mel (right)

I was off, no bye mum see you later. I was gone. The other two dogs were great, I ran around their garden, sniffed all around the bushes and trees, I was in doggy heaven. I was still rather nervous of these people and didn't want to eat my food. The lady even tried to get me to go upstairs to lay in the bedroom with her other dogs, but I just stood at the bottom of the stairs and said 'no, I'm not allowed up there'. In the end the lady came and slept on the settee to keep me company.

The reason I was with this lady was because there was going to be so much happening on the wedding day that Angela and David thought it wouldn't be fair for me to be ignored. Angela did not want to worry about me as she didn't have anyone to look after me; everybody would be at the wedding. Angela rang Guide Dogs for help in boarding me out. This is a service where there are volunteer boarders who will temporarily take in guide dogs and don't charge.

Now, you will have to understand that I wasn't at the wedding to tell you how it all went. By the time I'd finished listening to Angela and David telling the story of their wedding to whoever would listen though, I had a pretty good idea of what went on.

It was early in the morning when Angela got up, she had a lady coming to do her hair and make-up. Her daughter Clair arrived a little while later with her granddaughter Millie who was going to be a bridesmaid. Maria was up and in the kitchen finishing off the cooking. Maria barred anyone from going into the kitchen but Clair went in anyway and made some toast for Angela.

It was about eight in the morning when Angela's mobile went and it was her son Grant ringing from Thailand wishing her all the best for the day. It was hearing from her eldest son that set her off crying!

The wedding was to take place at eleven o'clock in the morning at Rochester Register Office. Angela put her dress on and then came out and paraded around showing herself off. David would later tell everybody 'she looked beautiful'.

Martin, Angela's second son, arrived in his car to take her to the Register Office. She was very nervous. There was a special moment between mother and son. They arrived at the Register Office and Angela was taken into a room to check over the paperwork. David was in another room at this point doing the same thing. The time came when Angela was walked down the aisle on the arm of her son who was giving her away.

The ceremony was short and soon over. Pictures were taken in and outside the Register Office and outside the nearby Rochester Castle. After all the pictures were taken it was then time to go to Mr Topes Restaurant where they had their wedding breakfast

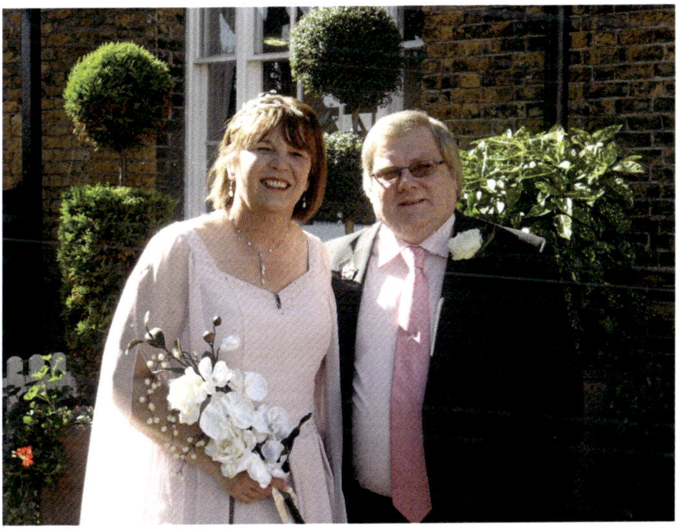

The new Mr & Mrs.

After the meal, everyone piled into their cars and left for the marriage blessing which was being held at Gillingham SNU Spiritualist Church in Canterbury Street. There were more guests arriving for the marriage blessing. The ceremony was really lovely. It was all about their beliefs in Spiritualism and the wordings were perfect for them.

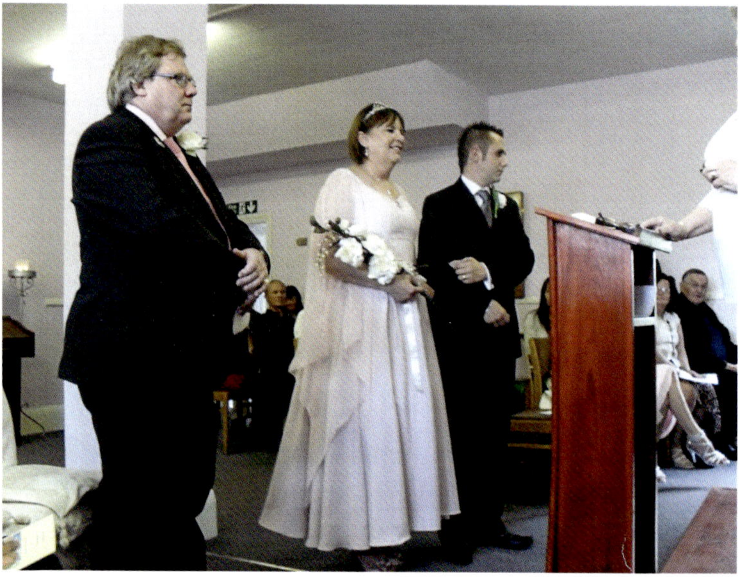

At their marriage blessing.

After the ceremony, more pictures were taken outside whilst inside, everyone mucked in together to get the hall ready for the celebrations. It was a wonderful tiring day and everybody enjoyed themselves. And I missed it all. All I was doing was being taken out for long walks in the woods, playing with my two new friends, sniffing anything and indeed anyone that came into my view, being fed and sleeping it all off. I think I got the best of the deal, don't you?

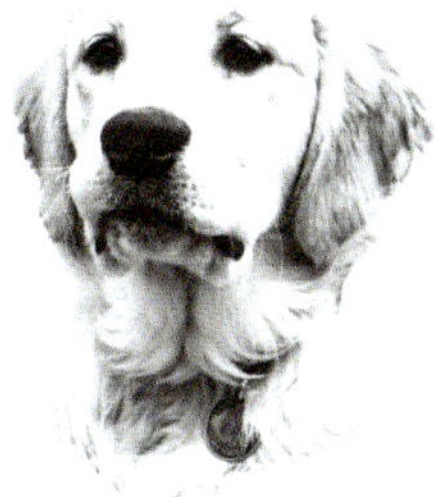

Chapter 11

Married Life

David finally moved in with Angela. It was on the Monday after the wedding when all the furniture and box shifting began. David hired a garage to put most of his stuff in as there was absolutely no room in the flat for all of his belongings. After about a week everything started to return to normal with the exception of one thing. David was now living with us.

We were still having people coming round to the flat every week doing their spiritual stuff. I was still sneaking up under the table to whoever would give me cuddles and treats but I had to make sure David couldn't see me either; there was an extra pair of eyes in the flat. David and Angela would take me out for long walks and I really liked this new life.

Angela and David didn't have a honeymoon at first. They saved up their money and paid to go on a coach trip to Chester and Wales. Once again I found my stuff being packed into the back of Clair's car (David didn't own a car then) and I stayed with Clair and her family. The family had two cats, Jagger and Cassie. Jagger didn't mind me much, sort of, but Cassie made it very clear that I wasn't welcome so she stayed out most of the time that I was there.

Clair's family love the outdoors. They go on long walks, bike rides, camping etc. Clair would always take me out for walks. I can remember two such excursions vividly, the memories will always stay with me.

The first occasion was when the family went for a long walk; a very long walk. At first when we started off I was all bouncy and excited, and when Clair let me off the lead, I would do a lot of running around. Then the lead went on and we went walking again. I began to think how far are we going? Time was going on and on and I was getting slower and slower. Instead of walking beside Clair I started to lag behind. Finally, we arrived home. I crawled indoors a few feet and collapsed and stayed there for the rest of the day. I didn't move, just slept.

The second memorable occasion was when Clair took her children to Mote Park in Maidstone and I went along too. Now, Mote Park has a lake and what are lake's made for, to jump in which was exactly what I did.

I went haring off once Clair unclipped me and I could hear this shouting 'Timber, stop!' well, I guess I must have needed my ears cleaning because I didn't hear that word 'stop!' It was glorious, feeling all this water around me. I was swimming around and then I started to notice that I couldn't feel the bottom anymore. Clair was calling me to come out, but I couldn't. I started to panic a bit wondering how I was going to get out. I started to swim towards a bridge and Clair managed to coax me to the side of the lake. She said for one minute she thought she would have to go into the water and get hold of me. I did get a telling off and was not allowed to go running around again in case I made another bee line for the water.

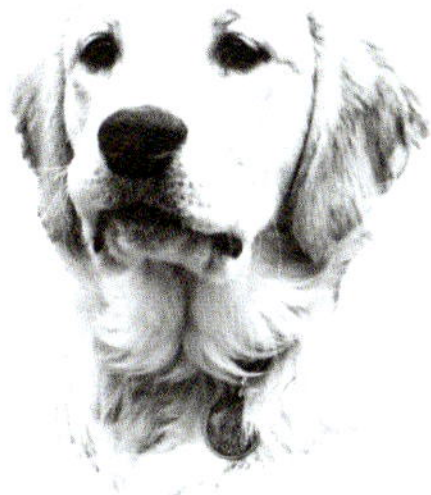

Chapter 12

Making me handsome

For those of you who do not what type of dog a Golden Retriever is I can tell you, I'm a hairy dog. I have a long fur coat that needs grooming every day or you can get away with every other day. I always knew when I was going to be groomed. Angela would go to the cupboard in the kitchen where she kept all my things, such as comb, brush, toothbrush and paste. I can hear you saying 'toothbrush?' Yes, toothbrush. My breath would really smell. I would know that as I would frequently get the comment 'oh Timber, go away your breath stinks'. Mind you it could be a bit difficult in trying to brush my teeth. I liked the taste of the toothpaste so much that I would lick it off before Angela could get the brush between my teeth.

Angela would then lay a special mat on the floor and place a towel over it. All she had to do was click her fingers and I was there. She would start by running her fingers through my coat. Just imagine somebody running their fingers through your hair and scalp, how does that feel? Good! She also did this to check if I had any ticks or fleas. She would then get the comb and comb my fur through. It's amazing the amount of fur that would come off me; a big pile, enough to knit a jumper.

After all that grooming, I would get a rub down with a brush and as a final touch she washed my face. The next stage of the grooming was my ears. Angela would get some wet cotton wool and root around inside them. They were always filthy and Angela would dread taking me to the Vet as he always picked on my ears saying they were dirty. Poor Angela. The final touch was the flea treatment which was placed under my collar so I couldn't get at it to lick it off.

After all of that Angela would give me a cuddle. When it was all finished, the first thing I wanted to do was go straight to the door so I could go outside and roll all over the dirt. Needless to say, she wouldn't let me out.

In spite of all her efforts in trying to keep my teeth clean, I had to go into the vets to be knocked out so that they could clean my teeth to get rid of all the plaque. I didn't really like that. It sort of put me out of action for a couple of days whilst the anaesthetic wore off.

Even with all of Angela's efforts to keep me tidy, I always somehow looked scruffy. I also got very hot during the summer months. Then Angela hit upon an idea of getting someone else to groom me and give my fur a good trim up. She found a lady who lived in Rainham and not only that, this lady was able to pick me up and drop me back home again afterwards. Her name was Carole.

She took me to her home where she had a special shed built at the end of the garden. I was washed, scrubbed, manicured and ears cleaned to within an inch of my life. Then she cut my hair. When Carole dropped me back home, I didn't look like me. I looked like a Labrador with a bushy tail and hairy ears. Angela was surprised at how I looked and I must say I did raise a few eyebrows when I was taken out to work. But I loved it.

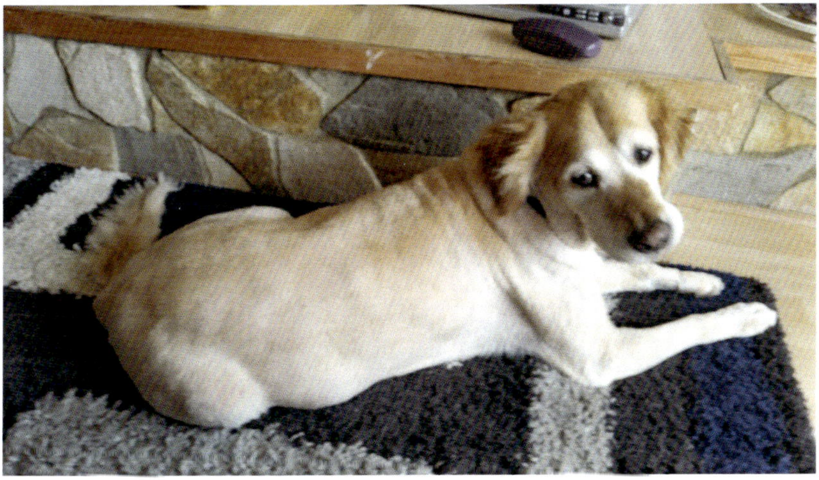

I've been groomed, this is me after my hair cut.

Every time I had my grooming done, I would go bouncing around as if I was a puppy again. It was so much cooler and a lot easier for Angela to groom me. Mind you I did have a slight complex at the beginning as I wondered what people would think of me, but they just said how handsome I was and then the old chest would puff out with me feeling so proud.

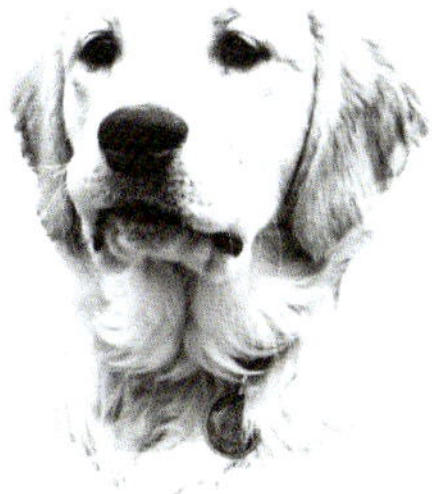

Chapter 13

Living on a building site

Before I get on with this particular story, I must tell you about two incidents that happened. Well, the first one was amusing to Angela but I didn't find it very funny. The second incident was quite serious and very upsetting. The first incident took place on a week day. David was at work and Angela decided that she needed to go to the local Tesco store which was just up the road from where we were living. Angela got me harnessed up and we left the house. She commanded me to go straight to the kerb first and then turn right. We walked up the road till it was time for us to cross. We made our way to the main crossing lights on the A2 where Angela gave the command 'find Tesco's'. Yes I'm that clever, I know where Tesco's is. When we got to a pedestrian crossing within Tesco's car park, I could hear a dog barking to my right. Me being nosey and wondering who it was that was trying to distract me, I just kept on looking to my right. Angela gave the command 'forward', she knew exactly what I was doing and was going to teach me a lesson. I walked forward, straight into a pole! Ouch! I could hear

Angela saying 'that should teach you a lesson, concentrate in the future', lesson learnt. If only I could have got my paw up to rub my head I would have done.

The serious incident occurred when Angela and I had been out for the day and were returning home from the town. We had got off the bus and we were about to cross a side road near the bus stop. Angela stopped at the kerb and as far as she was concerned there was no traffic about. When she stepped into the road, all of a sudden a car appeared from nowhere and ran over her foot. Angela was in shock. The driver got out of the car and started shouting at her; it didn't matter that I was there. He said that Angela had damaged his car and that he was going to sue her. When Angela said that he had run over her foot, he called her all the names under the sun, even though you could see the tyre marks on her suede shoes.

Angela was fuming and shaking all the way home. After we'd gone indoors and she had made sure that I was alright, Angela got straight on the phone to report the matter to the police. Apparently the man had already done so and they were aware of the incident. The police came round to take a statement. When Angela had finished, the police told her not to worry as the case would be dropped. I think they had a stern word to say to that driver when they realised that I was a guide dog.

Now back to the building site.

The Landlords decided that they were going to extend upstairs over the flat roof above our kitchen to make it into a proper self-contained flat. The work began just after Christmas of 2013. Then of course the rain came down and flooded the kitchen floor. I had to be moved into the living room as I couldn't stay in the kitchen. There were bricks missing from the side of the house in line with the roof and the cold air came blowing in through the gaps.

Each day the workmen turned up traipsing through the flat with their muddy boots. Angela became distressed with all the work that was going on and the loss of her privacy and having to keep cleaning the kitchen after the workmen had left, even after their half-hearted attempts at cleaning it themselves. The Landlords were not very helpful or understanding either. There were many heated words exchanged.

It was alright for David. He could leave the flat each day and go to work but Angela and I had to live in it. It got to the point when Angela said she had had enough of living where we were. She asked David if we could move.

During the month of February 2013 I began to notice that boxes were being packed and there was an air of excitement. Furniture was being moved into the front bedroom to make it easier to take it out to the moving van. On their last night, Angela and David slept on a mattress on the living room floor. Me, I was sleeping in my comfortable bed at Clair's house unaware of what was going on. It's a good life being a dog, sometimes!

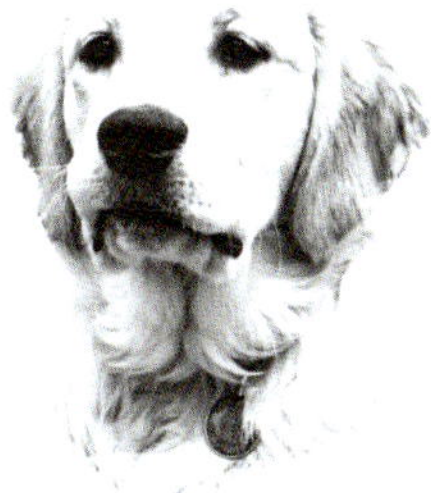

Chapter 14

My New Home and New Adventures

It was late afternoon when Clair and the children took me home. It was strange going in a different direction to the way we normally went but I was excited too. We arrived at the rear of the house; strange, I thought. Then we went up to the back gate and when Clair opened it I had a wonderful surprise; a real garden!

Oh wow, I was running around this new garden exploring everywhere. I even found a patch of long grass that I could roll around in. We went into the house and there were boxes everywhere. Angela was in the kitchen with Maria unpacking the pots and pans. Not only was there a garden, there were stairs in the house. It had been a few years since I'd seen stairs.

After everyone had left, David and Angela bought fish and chips and drank a toast with champagne to a new future.

It didn't take long to sort the house out and to get back into our normal routine.

What I haven't spoken to you about is the new beginnings with regards to Angela. I will have to back track here slightly as these changes started in the old flat in Twydall Lane.

Angela was running her circle one day when one of the students happened to comment about the Spiritual Centre closing down at The Oast House in Rainham. Maureen, the lady in charge, had decided that she couldn't run it anymore for personal reasons.

Whilst everyone was meditating, Angela's mind went into overdrive thinking about the Centre. Angela was having a conversation in her mind with her Spirit Guide. She was wondering whether she should approach Maureen about continuing to run the Centre after she had given it up.

After everyone had left for home, Angela phoned her husband David to run the idea by him. He told her to go for it and that he would support her in whatever she decided to do. Angela then rang Maureen, and put the suggestion to her and she gave her blessing. The Angel Messenger Centre was born.

So, not only was Angela sorting out her new house, she was sorting out her new Centre as well. We moved into the house on 3rd March 2013 and the Angel Messenger Centre was launched on 13th March 2013.

At the opening of the centre, Angela was feeling very excited and nervous at the same time; wondering if anyone was going to turn up. All the chairs were put in rows, the front table was dressed with candles and an Angel statue together with jugs of water and glasses. The medium for that first evening was David.

Some of Angela's friends arrived to help her. Kevin was a great support to Angela. He helped her in many ways because David was still going to work in London every day.

That first evening was a great success. There were over forty people in the hall. As for me, I enjoyed every minute of the fuss I was getting and of course, all the biscuit's!

We went to the Centre every Thursday. I really looked forward to going there, to meet new people, to be made a fuss of and for me to make a fuss of them. I could tell if someone was feeling sad, I would go up to them and sit by them just to say hello.

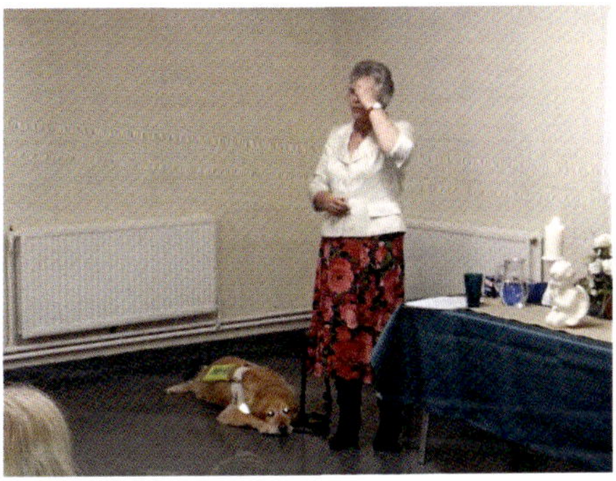

Angela talking to the audience.

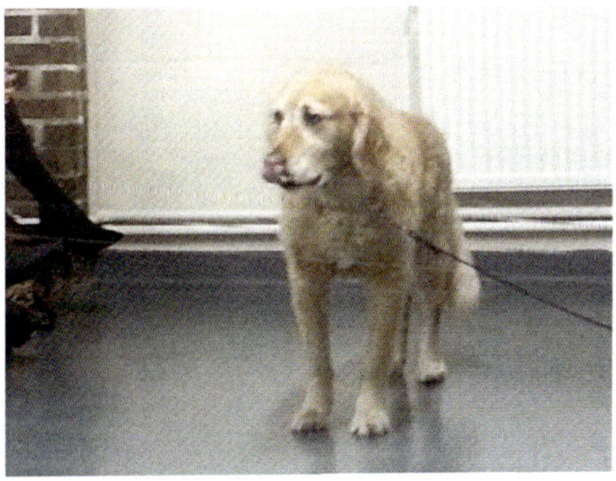

Getting ready to head for the kitchen!

Whilst the demonstration of mediumship was going on, I would just lie down beside Angela. Sometimes I would watch people or go to sleep. There was an occasion when a Medium named Jackie was right at the crucial point in her message. I sat up again and decided to put my two pence worth in. Of course the hall erupted into laughter. I always knew when the evening was coming to a close.

Angela would stand up to read the notices and I would hear someone get up and walk out to the kitchen to sort out the tea things.

Angela would then unhook my lead and I would be the first in the queue at the serving hatch when the doors were opened. Biscuits! There were times when Angela would make an announcement telling everyone not to feed me any. That didn't work. All I had to do was waggle my eye brows. It got them every time!

Angela held a lot of events at the Centre. She organised a Halloween Evening when everyone dressed up in appropriate costumes. The demonstration of Mediumship was given by Angela's good friends Josie and Trudy. This was followed by a fish and chip supper. After the supper, everybody went round the Oast House to link with Spirit. It was a wonderful evening. Angela held a Paranormal Evening, Psychic Fayres and raised money for three different charities, Guide Dogs being one of them. She also held an Animal Healing workshop with a gentleman called Henry Cummings. Angela even organised a day out to Avebury Stone Circle and Salisbury. Everybody enjoyed that. It was a great day, and nobody got left behind!

The Avebury trip was a great success. The weather was perfect. We arrived at Avebury and everybody went off to do their own thing. A lady named Marion held a meditation within the stone circle that everyone enjoyed. There was a tree on a hill where there were a lot of ribbons hanging in memory of loved ones who had passed or just to say 'I've been there'. Angela, David and I wandered around the stones. We had our pictures taken by various people. After all the walking around we ended up at the pub which was on the opposite side of the Stones. The pub was supposed to be haunted, but the only spirits in the place seemed to come out of bottles!

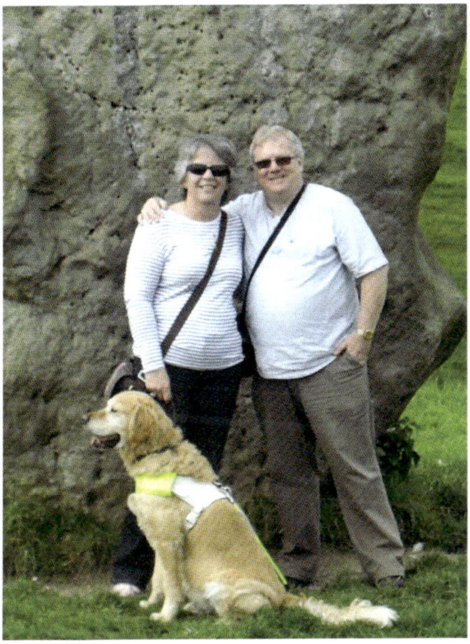

At Avebury Stone Circle.

After Avebury, we all got back onto the coach. Coach travel was new experience for me as I'd never been on a coach before that day. When we arrived in Salisbury, again everybody disappeared. Angela, David and I ended up in another pub; now is that telling you something?

I will tell you more about the Animal Healing workshop. In short, I loved it. Henry Cummings taught the students the benefits of spiritual healing for animals and showed them how to apply it. Early in the afternoon, a couple of dogs came into the hall to enable the students to practice healing on them. When it came to my turn, I went straight down onto the floor and it nearly sent me to sleep; it was heaven.

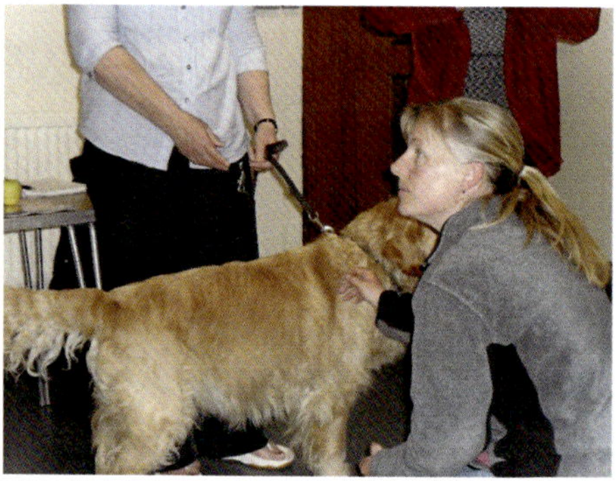

With Becky

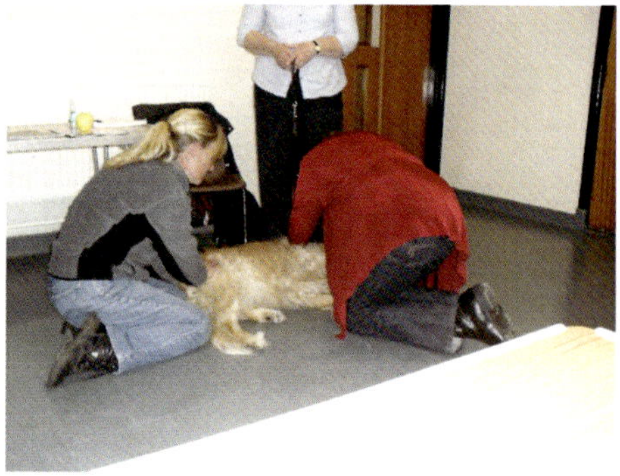

Out for the count!

It was later on in the afternoon when we packed everything away and trooped up to Angela's friend Becky's stable yard where she kept horses, goats and chickens. I was in my element. I kept running around the yard to say hello to all the horses. I even got up on my hind legs and touched noses with a couple of them to greet them properly.

I didn't like the goats much. You see, I'm a friendly sort of chap and would say hello to anyone. When I went up to this goat and got close to it, all of a sudden it head butted me! I was off. That taught me not to go near goats again. I went to the stable yard a few times after that; apart from the goats I loved it there. Not only the yard, I loved being with Becky too.

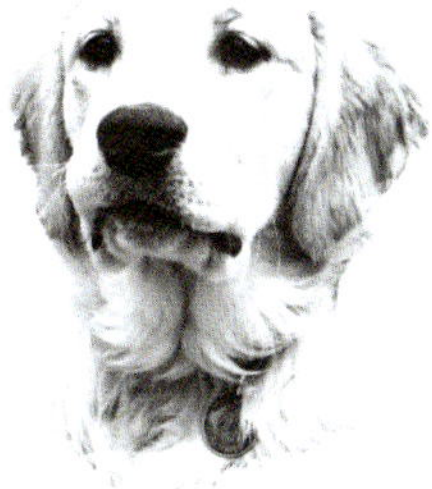

Chapter 15

Travel's and Troubles

It wasn't boring living with Angela and David. We did a lot of travelling around different places. Life got better once David bought a car. There was no more standing on cold wet platforms waiting for trains or standing at bus stops waiting for buses that invariably didn't arrive or were running late.

Angela and David would take me away on special occasions such as celebrating their wedding anniversaries. One particular year, they decided to go to The Walpole Bay Hotel in Cliftonville, (the posh part of Margate!) We were travelling on a train towards Margate, and I had adopted my usual position beneath the table out of the way. As the journey progressed Angela and David were approached by a young gentleman who had clearly imbibed a great deal of the juice of the hops. Swaying unsteadily clutching his can, he addressed Angela as follows 'ere, is that there one of 'em blind dogs?' Angela replied that actually I could see perfectly well and that it was she who had the eye sight problem! At this, the young gentleman staggered away down the coach gangway shaking his head and muttering to himself. Sometimes the ways of you humans are strange indeed.

We were now in the year 2014 having celebrated Christmas and the New Year. One thing I can say about Guy Fawkes and Christmas/New Year is that these occasions involve fireworks. I hated them! Indeed, I hated all loud noises. Angela tried several different remedies for this but she never found anything that worked. I was still petrified. There was one time when Angela and David had left me indoors whilst they popped out to the shops. Whilst they were out, I could hear in the distance a thunderstorm brewing somewhere and it was coming my way. When Angela and David came home, I was nowhere to be found. Angela was worried in case somehow I'd sneaked out of the house without them knowing. She was calling for me but I was under the bed in their bedroom and determined not to come out until the storm had definitely passed.

David's mother had a fall not long after this storm. At first it seemed that Eileen had just bruised her knee but eventually it turned into something more serious. After many trips to the doctors and hospitals, the surgeons decided that it would be best to amputate a couple of her toes that had turned gangrenous. She was admitted to Morriston hospital, Swansea, about May time.

What everybody thought was going to be a simple operation turned out to be really complicated. The surgeons decided that the gangrene was more serious and they took her leg off above the knee. Eileen didn't recover from this operation as well as she should have done so she remained in Swansea hospital under observation.

David had to travel either to Swansea or to his dad's home in the West Wales village of Aberarth to be with his parents and would leave Angela and me at home. David's dad Victor travelled every day the hundred and sixty miles round trip from Aberarth to Swansea and back to visit Eileen. She underwent another operation to take more of her leg off. I did get a chance to go and visit her in hospital once as I had been given special permission to enter the ward. This lovely surprise cheered Eileen up no end.

Eileen was in Swansea hospital for several months and her health was not improving. It was decided to transfer her to a hospital closer to her home and this made it a lot easier for David's dad Victor to visit her. Unfortunately, Eileen's condition worsened and it was in the month of August 2014 when she passed peacefully away.

Whilst Angela and David were worrying about mum, Angela was going through her own troubles. Angela started to have funny episodes when her vision would go black and white or become blurred. She also experienced a weird dizziness. We were in the Kent coastal town of Whitstable when I experienced first-hand one of Angela's attacks.

Angela was in a craft supply shop, when suddenly I could feel that something wasn't right with her. She became vacant (no change there some people might think), and I could feel her trembling through my guide dog harness. David came in to meet her and

Angela said 'I need to get out of here'. I could feel Angela walking erratically and she gave me the command to take her to a nearby seat. I was trying to support Angela while I was guiding her to the seat as I wasn't sure if she was going to fall. After sitting there for several minutes the episode passed.

When Angela spoke to her daughter Clair and her friend Maria about what had happened, they talked her into making an appointment to see the doctor. The doctor sent Angela for a CT scan and it was the day after David's mother passed away that Angela received the results.

I knew something was really wrong when Angela and David came home from the doctor's surgery. I could feel a tremendous sadness in the air. Neither of them was talking much to each other. Angela seemed to be in deep shock. It was whilst Angela was on the telephone talking to Clair that I found out what was wrong.

Angela told Clair that she had some bad news to tell her with regards to the recent CT scan. Angela told Clair that she had a tumour of the Meninges (a tumour on the lining of the brain). Angela had been told that such a tumour would probably turn out to be benign and could be operated on. When Angela came off the phone I could hear this howling sound coming from her bedroom. Angela was crying like I'd never heard her cry before. I just didn't know what to do to comfort her. All I could do was to sit or lie by her side just to let her know that I was there for her.

It was in September of 2014 when we were packing the car again to go on another journey. This journey was not a happy one. It was for the funeral of Eileen, David's mum. We arrived at a lovely B & B in West Wales and the owners made me very welcome. On the day of the funeral, David and Angela took me with them. We all climbed into the back of the undertaker's car. It was very uncomfortable for me as I couldn't sit in the front. I had to be squashed in the back with my nose pressing up against Angela. Angela couldn't move much to make it comfortable for me but she did try her best.

The crematorium was a stunning place as these places go. We all trooped into the waiting room while the other guests arrived and then we went into the chapel. There was an amazing view across the Welsh countryside from the huge window behind the altar. I also heard an amazing voice singing his heart out, it was David's.

We came back home to Kent. Waiting for Angela was a notification of an appointment see a Specialist at Darenth Valley Hospital in Dartford. Angela's doctor had pulled some strings to get her an early referral. After this Angela had to go for an MRI scan and then to see a Consultant at Kings College Hospital in London. The Consultant advised Angela to have the tumour removed as it was of a considerable size. It was about forty millimetres across.

We had a sombre Christmas that year but made the best of it. It was sombre because Angela didn't know if this was going to be her last Christmas together with the sadness of losing David's mum. Angela also received her operation date, twenty-first of January 2015; on her daughter Clair's birthday.

Before Angela underwent her surgery, she had to take Steroid tablets. Seeing these tablets reminded me about taking my own medicine. I had to take Thistleweed tablets every day to help my Liver function. Every morning Angela would call me to her and then open my mouth to place the tablets inside. She would hold my jaws together to make sure I swallowed the tablets but I had a trick up my paws. I would push the tablets to the side of my mouth and pretend that I'd swallowed them. When Angela wasn't looking I would spit them out. You should hear Angela when she found the tablet/s on the floor and I would get 'oh Timber!'

Just prior to Angela's operation, I reached another milestone in my life. Guide dogs usually work until they are between 10 and 13 years old depending on their condition. I was now almost 10 and it was time for me to hang up my harness. Luckily for me, Guide Dogs agreed that Angela and David could keep me as a pet. They even agreed to continue paying my vet bills and supplying me with food as I had been given to Angela under an older style of contract. So, I got to stay in my lovely home and I was also given a 'Retired Guide Dog' label for my lead. You'd be surprised at the places that this label got me into, even though I was retired!

Angela made arrangements for me to be looked after whilst she went into hospital to have her operation. Becky had very kindly offered to look after me. I knew I would be spoilt by her two daughters and her two dogs as well as by Becky and her husband. The great thing about staying with them was the huge field behind their home and Becky would let me loose in it. Not only in the field, Becky would take me to her stable yard. I would go around saying hello to the horses that were in their stables and then visit the ones that were out in the paddocks. I was still very wary of the goats; I had already learnt my lesson when I got head butted. When I saw Angela again I was so happy to see her. But, something was different about her; she seemed to be constantly tired and slept a lot and she'd complain about the pain in her neck and shoulder.

Maria had come to stay with us to look after Angela and David. She cooked the meals and kept Angela company when David had to go to work. There were times when Angela was telling Maria the story of her operation and she would begin to cry as she was very emotional.

I was cuddling close to Angela and eavesdropping on their conversation; you know me, always nosey. Angela told Maria:

On the day of the operation, Wednesday, we had to wait for the telephone call to say that there was a bed available for me before travelling up to the hospital at Denmark Hill, in London. The call came at about two in the afternoon. David and I looked at one another and hugged each other when I said 'this is it'.

We went to King's College Hospital by train and both of us were deep in our own thoughts. We didn't speak to each other much. We arrived at the hospital ward and were taken into a side ward where all of my details were noted down. The nurses explained what time I would probably be taken down to theatre the following day. David stayed with me for a while and then it was time for him to catch the train home.

During the evening, doctors came and went, the anaesthetist visited me and the Consultant came to check on me and explained that there would be three Surgeons attending the operation and then he went too. I was left alone for the rest of the night. Needless to say I didn't sleep very well as I had been told that I would be one of the first patients to be taken down to the theatre.

I was woken at six in the morning and was told to have a shower and put the lovely gown and socks on. I then waited and waited. My blood pressure was going up and up and the nurses kept coming into the room telling me not to worry and to try and get my blood pressure down. What a joke!

It was two in the afternoon when there was a commotion outside my room. The Orderlies had come to collect me. I was waiting outside the theatre doors when all of a sudden I felt a calm feeling come over me. Each of the three Surgeons came and introduced themselves and then I was left to the anaesthetist. I remember looking at the light just in front of me when all of a sudden it started to slide down the wall. I was asleep.

I was in theatre for some considerable time, I think about seven hours in all. Poor David and Clair, they were waiting for me upstairs and were frantic with worry. The fact that I was in the very same hospital where his late wife Val had been operated on for a malignant brain tumour was making it even harder for David.

I came up from theatre at about nine-thirty in the evening with my head bandaged up. It looked like a turban or as Clair said, a beehive. I was so happy to see David and Clair. David didn't need to say anything, I could see in his face the relief that I had pulled through. Mind you I was talking a lot of rubbish; no change there I hear you say!

I was told on the Friday (yes, only two days after the operation), that I could go home. That was quick! Although the food was disgusting, the doctors and staff had been great, except for the orderly who wheeled me down to the front entrance of the hospital. David went to fetch the car to pick me up and while he did so, the orderly just left me there at the hospital entrance all on my own! It was nice to be going back home though.

A few days later, I received a telephone call at about six in the evening from the hospital. I was very worried and wondered why they should be phoning me. I knew I would be going back to the hospital later that week to receive my biopsy results. The secretary on the other end of the phone told me my results there and then. She said that they had got the tumour out and tests had shown it to be benign. I just cried with relief. I was told that the surgeons had left a tiny node behind as it was attached to the main vein in my brain. If the surgeons had tried to remove it I could have suffered a massive stroke. The Surgeon did say that there was very little chance of the tumour ever growing back.

Angela made a remarkable recovery and was back on the rostrum working as a Spiritualist Medium six weeks after having her operation. I was sad about one thing though. It was at the Christmas get together at the Angel Messenger Centre prior to her operation when Angela announced that she would be stepping down from running the Centre that she had founded and would be handing it over to her friends Mel and Becky. Things were never quite the same after that. We did still go to the Centre but we were sitting amongst the congregation and it just didn't feel right.

Angela began to notice that I was having difficulties in jumping up into the back of the car and generally struggling getting up from the floor. I was now ten years old and age was starting to tell on my bones. Angela hit on the idea of buying me a dog ramp so that I could walk into the luggage space at the back of the car. Trying to get me to do this was another matter, however. This was where Guide Dogs came in. Angela was shown how to encourage me to walk on the ramp whilst it was lying flat on the floor with some treats on it. They then raised it up progressively until finally I could walk into the car. When the lady from guide dogs left, I said 'nope, not going to walk up it, treat or no treat'. In the end, David had to lift me in and out of the car and the ramp was never used for its intended purpose. That was much better.

It's now Christmas 2015 and I'm finding it increasingly difficult to continue writing this story. Angela and I are having a wonderful Christmas together. She and David are spoiling me rotten and we have our special grooming time together. Angela can sense that there is something wrong with me but she can't put her finger on it.

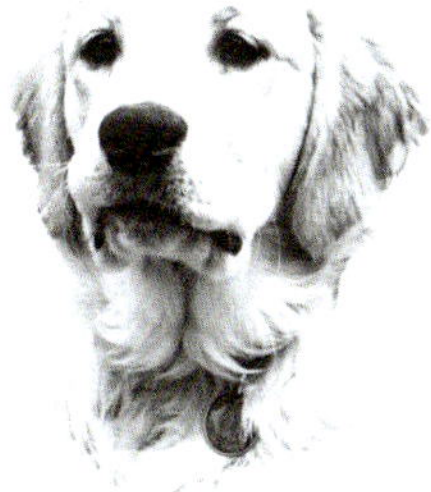

Chapter 16

Saying Goodbye

Hello everyone, this is Angela.

To continue writing Timber's Story from where he left off is one of the hardest things I've ever had to do.

It was December thirtieth 2015. David had got up to go downstairs and let Timber out into the garden to do his 'business'. Timber then came in and waited for David to open the cupboard door under the stairs where he knew his daily treat was kept. Timber took hold of the treat and went outside in the garden and lay down in his favourite place.

It was a little while after I'd got dressed that I came downstairs to greet Timber. Timber was still lying down outside. I took one look at him and thought that he didn't look right. I called to Timber to bring him back indoors but he just continued to look at me. I thought, okay, I'll give him another treat, but he didn't want to know. He struggled to get up and he just sat there watching me. This was definitely unusual.

I did manage to get Timber back indoors and I said to David that there was something wrong with him. I phoned the vet and explained Timber's symptoms and made an appointment for later that afternoon.

I went upstairs to do something but when I came back downstairs I could tell that something was seriously wrong with Timber. I laid down on the floor beside him talking to him. I hugged him and he felt cold and lifeless. I immediately shouted out to David that we had to take him to the vet's immediately. I phoned the vet's to tell them that we were on our way.

When we arrived at Wigmore Veterinary Surgery we were ushered straight into the examination room. The Vet was a lovely man who examined Timber and said that he was very anaemic and poorly. He said that he could have an internal bleed somewhere or he might have a problem with his spleen. If that was the case he could live without it if it was removed.

I was distraught to think my dear friend was having to undergo an operation so I got down on the floor to talk to him telling him that I loved him very much. I knew in my heart of hearts that I wouldn't be seeing my boy again.

It was about an hour after David and I got home from the vets when I received the dreaded phone call. Timber had cancer of the liver and there was no coming back from this. His condition was inoperable. I made the decision that it would be kinder to let him go. It broke my heart.

Timber taught me a lot. I'd never had a dog that was mine before. He taught me not to be afraid of dogs and to notice how wonderful they are. Each of them have their own unique characters. He was not only my guide dog he became my best friend. Timber touched the lives of everybody he came into contact with. Timber was loyal, (except that he would do anything for a biscuit), and watched my every movement to make sure I was safe. I loved him for that.

In commemoration of our life together, a memorial service for Timber was held at The Mind, Body and Spirit Centre next to the Medway Service area on the M2 motorway. I also wanted to write this book in Timber's memory. I hope it will raise awareness of Guide Dogs and the wonderful work that they do. Without Guide Dogs, people like me would find life very difficult. Timber gave me the confidence and the freedom to go out. He was the ice breaker in every situation. You could never be lonely when he was around.

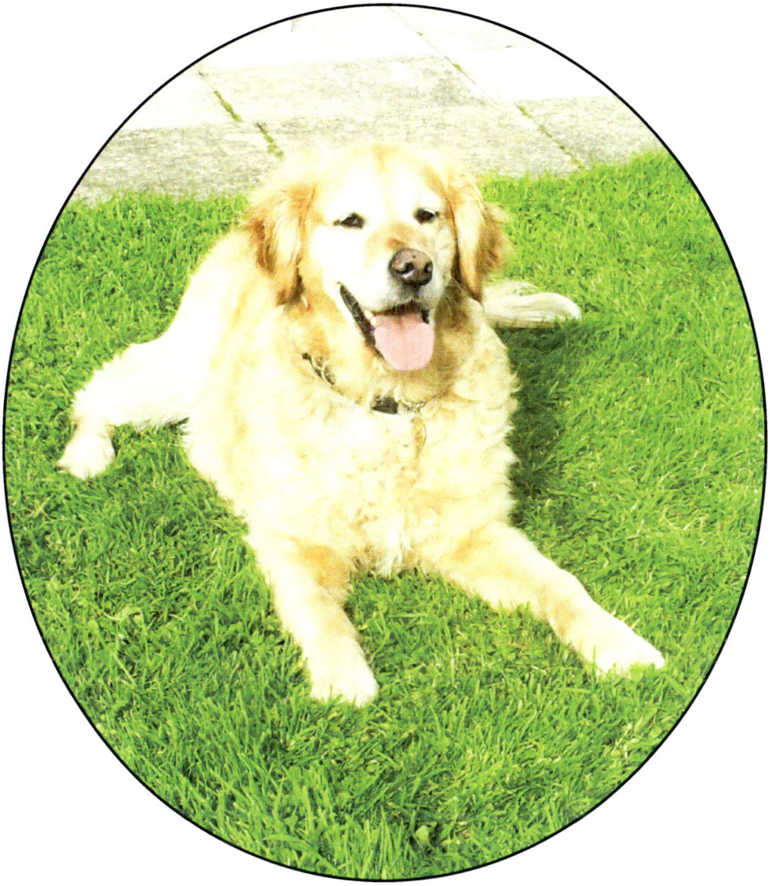

My boy Timber
(2005 - 2015)